S0-ADJ-819

WHAT PEOPLE ARE SAYING ABOUT CHAMPION MINDSET

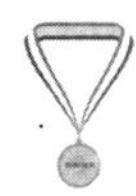

"Great book—a must for young competitors climbing that ladder to success. For me, extremely nostalgic journey of the past. Scott had and still has a great passion for ice skating. That's why he's one of the greats."

Ron Ludington
World & Olympic Coach
World Figure Skating Hall of Fame 1999

"I like the family and spiritual components throughout. Just when you think it's over for Scott Gregory, he finds a way to rally and reach new goals. The kid who grew up skating on a frozen lake in upstate New York took me on an inspiring journey all the way to the Olympics."

Peter Carruthers
1984 Olympic Silver Medalist

"Scott Gregory has written an inspiring, honest, and insightful account of his journey to the highest heights of athletic achievement. From his earliest days skating on a windy lake in upstate New York where he used his jacket as a sail, Scott describes a lifetime love for a sport that also dealt him some serious heartbreak. His will to persevere serves as an example to athletes young and old to never give up on your dreams, providing great perspective to anyone who thinks they have reached a dead-end. Scott learned how to implement values instilled in him from parents and coaches—positive attitude, hard work, focus, and faith—ultimately overcoming seemingly insurmountable obstacles and injuries to become a U.S. National Champion and two-time Olympian."

Paul Wylie
1992 Olympic Silver Medalist, Men's Figure Skating

"Even after a fifty-year involvement of all areas of skating, I was refreshed and inspired by reading about Scott's journey to his Olympic dream. While many dream about it, very few have the tenacity, courage, and passion to sacrifice so much, to endure through the painful experiences and hardships along the way. Scott shares about the price Olympic athletes pay as well as the victories and sweet rewards. As you read, you'll not only cheer for Scott but have a better understanding of anyone striving to reach their dream. For an athlete with a dream, for a parent or coach, this book is an inspiration . . . a must! I give this book a 10!"

JoJo Starbuck/Gertler
Two-time Olympian, World Bronze Medallist
and U.S. Figure Skating Hall of Famer

"This book is very inspirational for any athlete, not just figure skaters. In fact, the story of struggle and determination is relevant to all realms of life. Anybody who has tried their best and been sabotaged by circumstances beyond their control would benefit from reading *Champion Mindset*."

Karen Cover
World Figure Skating Museum & Hall of Fame Archivist

"Throughout history we see man's natural ability to persevere through hardships and adversity to survive and to achieve the improbable. This book not only captures the mindset of a champion skater and his tenacious attitude through many intense years of training but also speaks of how necessary faith, family, and friendships were to reaching his lifelong goals. As a parent of a young skater, I found *Champion Mindset* to be a superb example of the courage, perseverance, and passion that serious athletes must have to reach their goals. I read this book with my daughter, and we both found it difficult to put down. Written in a very encouraging and uplifting way, these pages provide an ideal touchstone for any athlete determined to begin a journey to achieve."

Heidi Morris
Parent of a young athlete

Champion Mindset

Refusing to Give Up Your Dreams

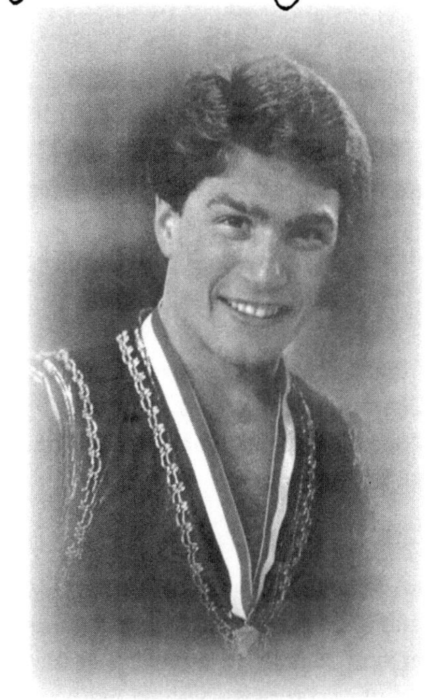

Scott Gregory

with Diane Cook

How one Olympian found the courage and inspiration to persevere through devastating setbacks. This story will compel kids and their parents to ignite the winner inside.

CHAMPION MINDSET
Refusing to Give Up Your Dreams

Copyright © 2010 Scott Gregory
ISBN 978-1-886068-41-4
Library of Congress Control Number: 2010932472

Published by Fruitbearer Publishing, LLC
P.O. Box 777 • Georgetown, DE 19947
(302) 856-6649 • FAX (302) 856-7742
www.fruitbearer.com • info@fruitbearer.com

Cover and graphic design by Candy Abbott
Edited by Fran D. Lowe

Cover photo of Scott Gregory by Howey Caufman from 1987 U. S. Figure Skating Championships (original photo with Suzanne Semanick, U. S. Senior Dance Champions, published on the cover of the April 1987 *Skating* magazine)

All rights reserved. No part of this publication may be reproduced, stored in a retrieval system, or transmitted in any form or by any means—electronic, mechanical, photocopy, recording, or any other—except for brief quotations in printed reviews, without the prior permission of the publisher or author, except as provided by USA copyright law.

Printed in the United States of America

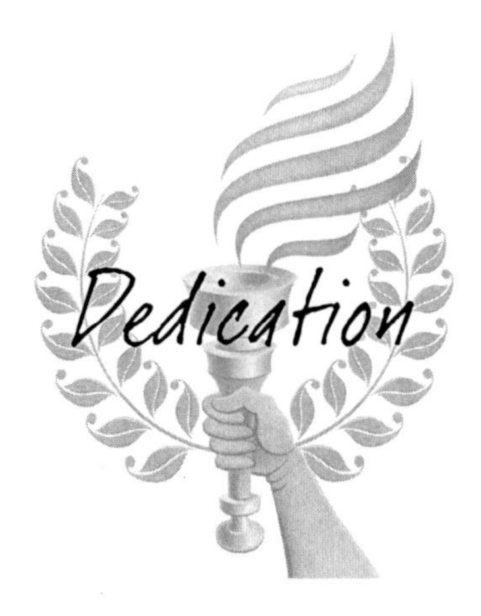

Dedication

To Mom and Dad, I will never forget my childhood memories of growing up on Skaneateles Lake. In fact, I cherish to this day those early times of skating on the frozen lake. All the great and not so great trips to competitions, shows, and tours are forever etched in a beautiful spot in my mind. You always showed me right from wrong through your guiding care. Reliving those years through these pages, helps me appreciate just how deep your love for me is and realize how often I took it for granted. Without your unconditional love, support, and sacrifices, my dreams could not have come true. I thank you from the depths of my heart.

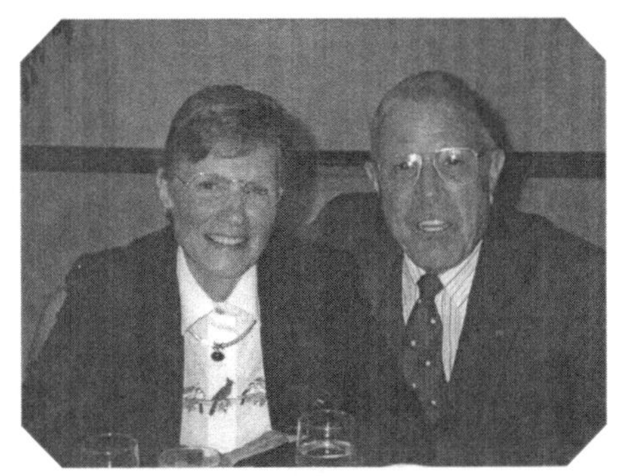

Mom and Dad, Bill and Bayne Gregory
1998

Contents

Champion Mindset

Refusing to Give Up Your Dreams

Chapter 1

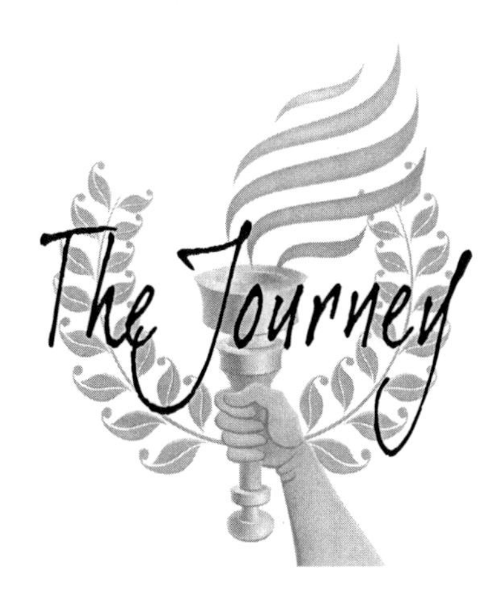

The Journey

"Sir?" A woman's soft voice drew me out of a deep sleep. "Sir, we're about to land. We have to sit you up now."

Pain shot through my lower extremities as the flight attendant gently raised my seat back. *Wow! That hurts.* I instinctively held my breath as I tried to resist the groans and grunts pushing through my vocal chords. I blinked back tears that threatened to roll down my cheeks.

"A wheelchair will be waiting for you at the gate."

"Thank you," I gritted. Nodding my head was too painful.

"Can I get you anything?"

"A new back?" I was trying to be funny, but it wasn't working.

She knelt beside my seat in the first-class cabin. "You will be one of the last off the plane."

"Could you put this back in my skate bag?" I asked as I handed her my Walkman and headset.

She stood and removed the red-and-blue bag sporting a white USA figure skating emblem on it from the overhead bin. Unzipping it, she placed the tape player inside.

"Your bag says 'World Team.' How long have you been skating?"

"Seriously, since I was eleven," I replied, wondering if I would ever be on the ice again. This wasn't how I had planned to return from an international competition.

"You look familiar," she said, taking the blanket that had covered me during the eight-hour flight home. "Are you famous? Should I know you?"

I would have laughed if it didn't hurt so much. "Sort of, but not really."

"Oh," she replied, obviously more puzzled than ever. Further questions were interrupted by the flight crew's call to their seats because the plane was landing.

Moments later, the jumbo jet's huge wheels contacted with the runway. Even though my airline pilot dad would have called this a smooth landing, every bump jarred my injured back. How could this have happened just two months before the U. S. National Figure Skating Championships, and in an Olympic year at that? I was so close! Was this the end of my sixteen-year struggle?

It couldn't be over! I was only twenty-eight!

"Tough break, Scott," one of the U. S. competitors commented as he inched by me on his way to the aircraft's front exit.

"I hope we'll see you at Nationals in February," his petite brunette partner said on her way out.

"Did you get any rest?" my partner, Suzy Semanick, asked as she slipped into the seat across the aisle, waiting with me until the wheelchair came. Robbie Kaine, one of my coaches, slid into the seat behind me.

"Yeah," I muttered. "I'm sorry, Suzy. This whole trip was a waste."

"Stop saying that!" she said. I could see her getting angry again. "None of us planned for this to happen. We've just got to get you home to a doctor to see what's going on. You'll be back on your feet in no time."

"Your ride is here." The flight attendant stepped aside while an airport employee rolled one of those ugly-looking wheelchairs toward me.

"This isn't going to be easy," I said. I tried to stand but couldn't.

Robbie reached over the top of the seat and started lifting me from behind while I tried to steady myself by pushing up on the chair arms. The flight attendant pushed the chair in at an angle while Robbie pivoted my tensed body toward it. As my body settled in the worn sling seat and back, I tried to stifle the noise that stuck in my throat. I hit my back too hard—way too hard. It hurt more this time: I was in literal agony.

Suzy moved around to the front and lifted my feet onto the running board so we could finally deplane. Puzzled stares followed us as Suzy wheeled me down the walkway. I suppose we looked rather odd—a young guy holding onto a skate bag as if his life depended on it while a gorgeous blonde pushed him through the crowded Philadelphia International

Airport. We probably looked vaguely familiar to sports fans, but without the familiar red, white, and blue USA apparel they most likely couldn't place us.

I was glad because I hated being seen like this—helpless, hurting, and perhaps at the end of my career. Thoughts of future competitions had given way to mind-numbing pain. My dad told me years ago that injuries never come at a convenient time, and he was right. I just wondered if I could bounce back from this setback in time.

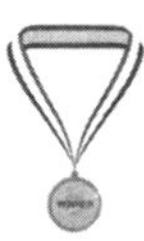

I had experienced many hindrances during my seventeen-year journey in the world of amateur ice skating, but I could never imagine doing anything different. Even as a young boy, I knew no fear; in fact, I was always the first to accept a dare and rush in without considering the consequences. The youngest son of Bill and Bayne Gregory, I was born in 1959 in the small town of Skaneateles, snuggled in central New York's Finger Lakes region. Glacier-formed lakes looked like God just scooped His curled fingers into the landscape, leaving rolling hills and huge valleys filled with water.

Mom was an elementary school physical education teacher, and Dad was a local businessman and airline pilot who flew with the Air National Guard. My sister, Heather, was a year older than me; and my brother, Bill Jr., nicknamed "Bee Gee," was three years older.

Skaneateles was a great place to grow up because it was literally a kid's paradise. Sailing, swimming, boating, and water skiing filled my time in the summer; but during the bitterly cold central New York winters, the lake froze. Staying inside where it was warm wasn't an option for an adventurous kid like me, so I roamed outside as often as my mother would let me. It was out there that I entered the magical world of ice.

I can't say when I first became aware of the lake just ten feet from my back door. My favorite family picture was me at eight years old, well-bundled in a snow suit, hat, mittens, and boots. I was standing on crackled black ice surrounded by dusty snow mounds, with the shoreline and our house in the background. All this, along with the bitter cold, was my idea of an awesome time.

Even though we called it "black" ice, it is actually totally clear. In fact, you can look down through this kind of ice as if you were peering through a magnifying glass and see everything close up—even the rocks at the bottom of the lake and fish swimming by. It's like nature's aquarium.

Living on the lake meant getting to know your neighbors really well, especially those who had neat toys like my Uncle Jack. His red two-seater ice boat was a people magnet. Ice boats, which look like sailboats with sled runners, are fun because they catch the wind and sail across the frozen lake at phenomenal speeds.

When Uncle Jack sailed by, lakeside families knew that it was time to come out and play. Like the Pied Piper, he'd entice our neighbors outside in their skates or boots within moments to enjoy an impromptu block party on ice. The lucky ones got to ride on the ice boat. Thrilled by the prospect of the freedom of gliding on the ice and feeling the wind in my face, I *had* to be first in line.

Winters in Skaneateles were brutal, especially the one in 1966. Even though I was only seven years old that year, I still remember the enormous amount of snow piled up over our cars and blocking the entrances to our homes. Our family could barely get out of our house for two days because the roads left unplowed kept us snowbound.

So my siblings and I sat at the window and watched the snow fall, wondering when we could venture into the wonderland that awaited us. Once the weather cleared, it didn't take long for us to escape from our captivity and engage in adventures that could only happen outside. We were so busy sledding, building forts, and pummeling each other with snowballs that the cold meant nothing to us. Our world revolved around the possible intriguing shapes that we could mold from the icy wonders at our fingertips. Early dusk drove us inside, where warm meals and mugs of hot chocolate revived us, stoking our desire to go out and have fun in the ice and snow again and again.

We didn't need a blizzard to give us clearance to skate on the lake. All we needed was a cold spell sufficient to freeze the water for a week or more. By then, the foot-thick ice was cold, cold, cold and ready for fun.

Designed for beginners, my first pair of skates (double runners) strapped onto my snow boots and looked more like butter knives. They weren't good for much more than walking on the ice, so I wanted more.

I yearned to glide on the ice like the bigger kids, hockey players, and speed skaters. When I was nine years old, I decided to take matters into my own hands. Knowing there just had to be some real skates in the house somewhere, I looked for weeks and weeks. I was getting angrier at every failed effort, until the day I attacked the hall closet.

I opened the tall wooden door and carefully eyed the boxes piled behind heavy coats and jackets. Pushing through this fabric jungle and wading past the mountain of rubber boots, hockey sticks, and umbrellas, I eyed a tattered-looking box in the back corner. Could this be the treasure that had eluded me for so long?

Dropping to my knees, I gently picked up the box. After brushing the dust off of the lid, I carefully removed it from the base. There they were—the perfect skates, laying in a bed of tattered tissue paper and just waiting to be rescued. I didn't see worn black-and-brown leather on top of rusted but sturdy blades; instead, I saw my ticket to freedom on the ice.

I lifted my treasure from the box and tugged on the laces. Although well-worn and frayed, they were still strong. Setting the box aside, I took the right skate and gingerly pushed my foot inside. It almost fit.

"Extra socks! That's what I need!" I shouted, tossing the skates back into their battered cardboard box and running to my bedroom. "Mom! Where are my heavy socks?"

"They should be in your top drawer." Her voice wafted from the other side of the house. Opening the dresser drawer, I found the socks and counted the ones I would need.

"One, two, three! That should do it." I pushed the drawer shut with an extra flourish, sat on my bed, and flipped off my shoes. With great anticipation, I fit sock over sock until my toes were so cramped that I couldn't even wiggle them.

Leaving my street shoes behind, I padded down the steps to the open closet. Sitting on the floor, I reverently removed the skate from its box and slipped it on my fully-padded foot. My foot slid inside as though this was the home it had been waiting for forever. I pulled the laces as tight as I could and then looped them around the top twice before tying the final knot. I repeated the ritual with the left skate and then leaned back on both hands to admire my handiwork.

"They look good," I said, gazing upon the grown-up sized, two-tone leather skates. Then I grabbed the closet doorknob and pulled myself up, my heart pounding with excitement. I couldn't believe my luck: I was ready to try the ice with these great new weapons. Even these ancient hockey skates could outperform my butter knives in a heartbeat.

I heard my mother puttering around in the kitchen. My older brother and sister were out with their friends. After donning my coat, hat, scarf, and gloves, I wobbled into the hall and out the door to the frozen lake.

The icy Skaneateles wind whooshed past me as I slammed the door shut. The ten feet between the door and the lake seemed like a hundred yards as I clomped through twelve-inch snowdrifts. With no hand-holds, I crawled as far as I walked. The hockey skates and triple pairs of socks added extra weight, but I was determined to reach the ice, no matter what.

Though it seemed like hours, I reached a barrier about five minutes later. Lake winds had pushed snow and ice to the water's edge, creating Everest-like drifts. They were probably two and a half feet high, but they seemed like mountains to me. On hands and knees, I worked my way to the top. I don't know that any mountain climber could have been prouder than I was the moment I reached the peak.

After relishing my victory for a moment, I discovered an even greater challenge. Now that I was at the top, I had to find a way to get to the bottom! As I sat down to ponder my dilemma, I suddenly found myself sliding toward the frozen ice—a human bobsled with only my bottom and legs to guide me. Gaining speed, my slide to the bottom of the mound propelled me a few feet onto the ice.

Looking around to see if anyone had observed my clumsy entrance, I was relieved to find that I was alone. Standing was the next problem I had to overcome. Cautiously, I placed my right foot in a standing position, then my left. Before I could get my left foot in place, *kaboom!* My right foot had slid out from under me!

Another half hour must have passed while I tried to get both feet on the ice at the same time, but my persistence finally paid off. At last, I managed to stand. The first goal was achieved, now onto number two. Taking one deep breath to rouse my courage, I slid off with my right foot and then followed with my left. Much to my delight, I was moving!

Freedom is expressed in many ways. For me, it was feeling the wind rush past me like the times I was on Uncle Jack's ice boat. Only this time, it was better because my body, which was out of control, was now in control. I was making this remarkable thing happen in a grand new way. This single action initiated me into the magic of the ice. I was at one with the lake, and a new journey had begun.

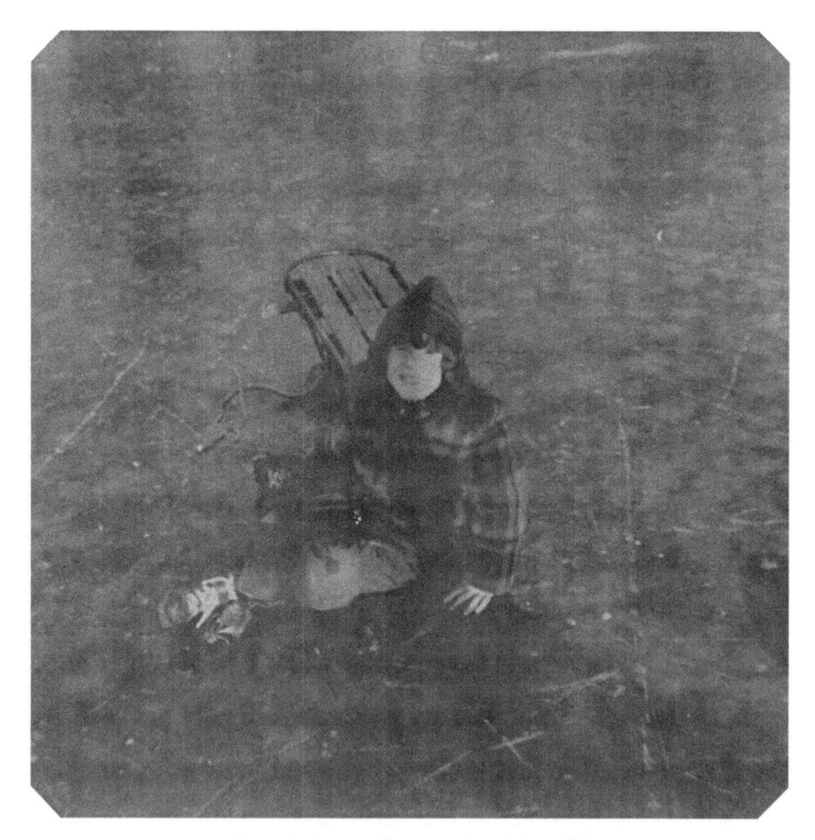

My early days on Skaneateles Lake, 1966

Chapter 2

A Brave New World

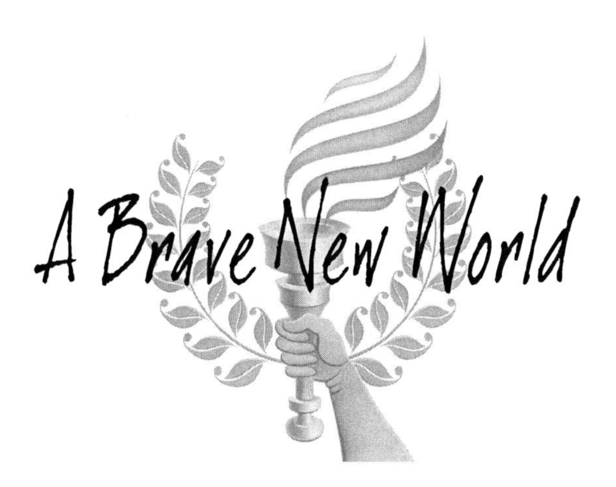

My fondest memories on the lake were those times when I would go out alone and experience the ice. I loved skittering across the lake, so I developed all sorts of techniques for wind propulsion, especially on gusty days. Sometimes I would lean into the wind and let it push me backwards. When I felt especially inventive, I would take a towel and tie it around my waist. Then I would take a corner of the towel in each hand and stretch my arms out to become a human mast to my terry-cloth sail. And then there were times when I would convert my sled into a mini ice boat. With me serving again as the mast, I would tie both ends of the towel to the sled's steering mechanism. Then I would sit on the sled with my feet against my makeshift wheel while I held the other corners of the towel in each hand. Its effectiveness was incredible, whisking me across the ice at incomprehensible speed. I was addicted to the thrill of it all.

For two winters, the lake served as my rink, the wind as my companion, and personal imagination as my motivator. This continued until 1971, when some of my mother's friends decided that we needed a figure skating club to use our town's newly built open-air rink. So, naturally she was on the committee that founded and formed the Skaneateles Figure Skating Club. I was eleven years old at the time.

It was mid-October, and all that my friends were talking about was which super-hero they were going to be for Halloween. I preferred my homemade hobo costume—Dad's oversized gardening shirt and pants made to fit me with a well-stuffed pillow. The dirtier and tattier the better was all I was thinking about when we sat down to eat my least favorite dinner menu.

I stuffed a fork full of spinach into my mouth all at once, careful to chew it well so I wouldn't choke on it like I did the last time Mom served it. I figured that the taste wouldn't linger if I chewed it fast and first, and then followed it with a generous swig of milk.

"Mom, where are Dad's old pants I wore last year for my hobo costume?" I asked in mid-chew.

"Check the garage," she replied, "and don't talk with your mouth full."

I took my milk swig before forming my next question, but Heather beat me to the punch.

"When are you starting the skating club?" Her question was innocent enough, but I was more interested in my costume.

"November," Mom said. "I've signed you kids up for eight group lessons to see how you like it."

"It sounds like fun," Heather replied, looking at Bee Gee for support.

"Yeah," he replied, less than enthusiastically. "Fun . . ."

"Do we have to take lessons with Scott?" That was the mantra around the house. Don't get me wrong. My brother and sister were cool, but as the youngest, I was definitely a third wheel.

"No," Mom replied, "He'll be in a different group."

"Now back to my costume," I announced, not giving the lessons another thought until after Halloween.

But my costume was definitely not a priority for the rest of the family at dinner that night. It turned out to be a discussion about preparations for the skate club, the new coach that the city's parks and recreation department hired, and how long the rink would be open. Meanwhile, I was developing my strategy for the year and wondering if Mom would miss her broom handle if I used it for my hobo sack, which I planned to fill with candy.

The excitement of Halloween came and went. All too soon, it was time to meet our eight-lesson obligation to help get the Skaneateles Figure Skating Club off its feet. Our newly built rink was an outdoor structure, open on three sides with one roofed warming room and lights. It was cold, almost as cold as the lake.

Of course, my dad's hockey skates wouldn't work for rink skating, so my mom bought me my first real skates—black CCM's, complete with a toe pick. With these beginner's skates that were flimsy and floppy, it was like skating with paper boots and a real cheap blade, but at least they fit my feet. They were my first special skates, so I was proud of them. Not only did I have my CCM's, but I also got my own skate bag filled with skate guards, a towel to wipe off the blades so they wouldn't rust, and everything else I needed.

From that point on, ice skating dominated my thoughts, and I often doodled their shapes in my notebook margins. In one of my art classes, we were told to draw a life shield, which was supposed to have four interest points that represented the artist on the front. I'm still surprised by the way it connected together. My shield had an ice skate with the laces connecting to my stereo, a mountain, and a pond with me skating on it. Little did I know at the time that I would still have the drawing after I was married, grown, and blessed with a daughter of my own.

Despite the coolness of my first "fit-my-foot" skates and accessories, I was only mildly interested in the club until the close of the first lesson. Then something special happened under the gentle tutelage of my first coach, Michael Paikin, who introduced me to discipline on the ice. It was no longer enough to experience freedom and speed; now it was time to discover the art of the ice.

Michael's approach was organized and required skill, training, and lots of practice. My years on the lake had helped me gain balance and a love for speed, so it didn't take long for me to be one of the fastest in my age group. A girl named Carey came in a close second.

"Hey, Carey," I yelled across the ice one day. I was ready for my favorite move. "Let's do a 'shoot the duck.'"

She left the gaggle of girls in the corner and skated toward me, hand extended. I grabbed her right hand, and we stroked to get up speed. Then we squatted down on our left legs with our right legs extended out in front. Leaning our upper bodies way forward, we shifted our weight and grabbed our left knees, bending forward as far as we could go. We were human go-carts, close to the ice with our momentum carrying us until Carey lost her balance. Both of us toppled onto the ice, laughing the whole time.

"Scott!" I heard my coach calling my name across the rink. "Come here." I left Cary and glided effortlessly over to Michael, who was talking to my mom.

"Yeah, Coach?"

"Your six weeks with the group are almost over," he said. "How would you like to take private lessons?"

"What happens in private lessons?"

"You'll learn to do school figures and more advanced jumps, spins, and some dance patterns. You'll have one-on-one time to accelerate your skating. In other words, you'll learn a lot faster. Are you up for it?"

I could feel my heart pounding in my ears. Something started to break loose: my special love for skating.

"Mom, could I?"

A quirky smile played on her lips as she nodded her head.

"When do I start?"

"Next Tuesday, six o'clock," Michael said. "Be here and ready to go."

"Sure," I replied. "I can do that."

Mom nodded at Michael. "Come on, Scott, let's go."

"Now?"

"Yes," she said in her best teacher voice. "You have homework to finish."

I groaned on the outside, but inside I was pleased with this new turn of events. Something special was happening, and I liked it.

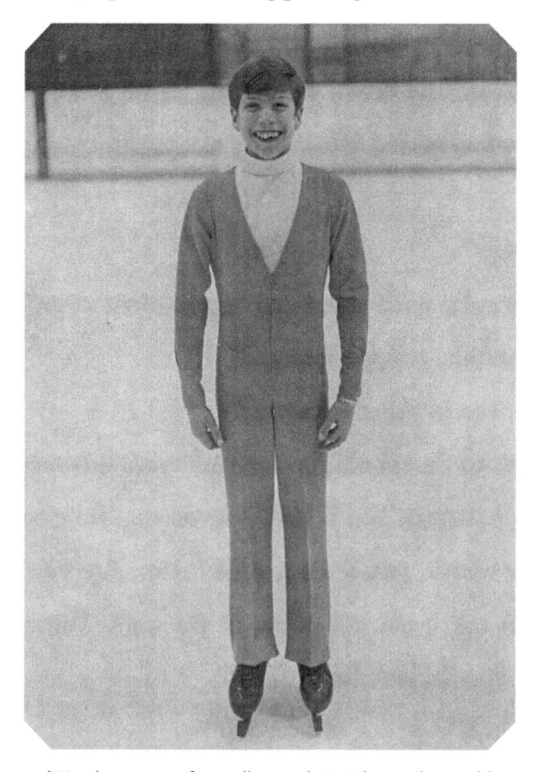

At twelve years of age, I'm ready to take on the world.

Chapter 3

Private Lessons

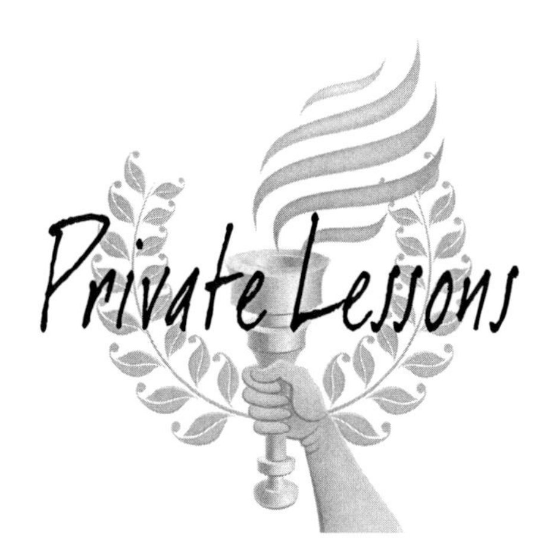

I started private lessons the next week. We often began our sessions with school figures, also known as figure eights. That meant we had to skate in perfect circles and then go back and retrace the etched pattern three times without going off the original line. This taught control and forced us to concentrate as we learned the body movements required for this level of precision. While some found this boring, I did not. The rink remained quiet, and the soft hissing of a dozen skaters' blades connecting with the ice relaxed me, allowing me to enjoy the challenge, especially when I did it right.

Since the International Skating Union no longer requires figures in competition, this part of the sport may seem archaic. But at the time, it served as a good training tool for me.

I worked both at freestyle skating and ice dancing during these first months with Coach Paikin. He taught me a few basic dances like the

Dutch Waltz, Canasta Tango, and Swing Dance. I had also learned all my single jumps and was starting to do a one-and-a-half rotation in a jump called the Axel.

I was progressing well, but I didn't know how well until one lesson day when I was practicing my figures. The rink was so quiet that all I could hear was the crisp sound of blades on ice.

"Hey, Scott!"

"Yeah, coach?" I answered, my voice hushed.

"Come here a minute."

I stopped my circles and glided over to him, executing a perfect stop.

"Scott, I'm teaching at R.I.T.'s summer skating camp this year."

I must have looked puzzled because he laughed. "R.I.T. is the Rochester Institute of Technology. They have excellent ice skating facilities there and open it up as a summer camp for skaters of all ages. You jump well, your spins are good, and I think you're ready for the summer camp experience. Do you want to give R.I.T. a try?"

"Sure, coach." I hesitated. "I'll have to ask my parents."

His quiet smile released me from our conversation, so I returned to my figures. My lesson seemed to drag on forever because I could hardly wait to get home that night. I really wanted this, but now all I had to do was convince my parents. They'd been pretty cool about my skating, especially since my grades were improving, but this was something extra. Little did I know that Coach Paikin had already talked to them.

Dad picked me up on his way home from work. He didn't have much to say, and I was too preoccupied with what kind of deal I should offer if they let me go to R.I.T.

"Wash up for supper," Mom said as we walked into the kitchen from the garage.

"Mom, I need to talk to you and Dad." I was ready to negotiate, but Mom wouldn't hear of it.

"We'll talk after dinner. How much homework do you have?"

"Just math," I replied, a bit disgruntled about having to wait.

For the most part, Heather and Bee Gee carried the conversation during dinner. At least we were eating food I liked—baked chicken, mashed potatoes and gravy, green beans, and hot rolls.

I tried to pick at my food, but it was too good to ignore. Then I got the idea that if I ate really fast, we'd get through dinner so I could talk them into the camp.

"Slow down, Scott," Mom said as she caught me shoveling a huge mound of mashed potatoes in my mouth.

I started to form a word, but my mouth was kind of stuck; so I just nodded my head and chewed slower. By the time I slowed down enough to catch up, supper was over, and it was time for us to talk.

Mom and Dad were seated on the sofa, and I sat in the matching armchair off to the side. Dancing flames from the fireplace added to the room's warmth. An occasional well-burnt falling log emitted a short shower of sparks, releasing a fragrance that triggers good memories of hearth and home for me even today.

I cleared my throat as I prepared to speak. "Um, Mom and Dad, I think Coach Paikin may be speaking to you sometime soon."

"Oh?" Dad leaned forward. "Are you in trouble or something?"

"No!" I couldn't believe my dad would think that. He knew how much I loved skating, didn't he? "Um, well, um, the coach thinks I should go to summer ice skating camp in Rochester, and so do I!" I said this so fast that I could barely understand myself. "Um, I mean—"

Mom burst out laughing.

"Bayne, stop it!" Dad said, laughing almost as hard as she was.

"What's so funny?" By this time, I was starting to get mad.

"Honey, Coach Paikin talked to us before he even mentioned it to you. We've already said yes. You're going."

I fell back into the chair, groaning. All that worrying was for nothing!

"Now, go do your homework," Mom said quietly. "And I'm glad you're doing so well."

"Thanks, Mom," I said as I stood up and started to leave the room. Then before I realized that I had changed direction, I was hugging them both. "You're the best."

"All right, now get upstairs, and do your homework," Mom said as I turned away and bounded up to my room, two steps at a time.

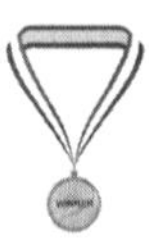

Spring gave way to summer, and before I knew it, I was at camp. Rochester Institute of Technology was an entirely different world; in fact, it was like visiting Disney World for the first time. There were plenty of good skaters. I watched them for hours, doing doubles and triples. They were doing all these complicated moves, and I was just learning the singles.

The instructor's command drew me away from the boards onto the ice with the other rookies. "Let me see what you've got," he said as I came to the center, joining my fellow skaters. Four older girls moved off center as I took my position.

"Okay, now try this," he said after handing his clipboard to an assistant. He executed a perfect Axel.

Up till now, I had been involved at the beginning stages of my Axel training with Coach Paikin. There was just something I wasn't getting, however; so I watched this instructor closely, registering his posture, weight distribution, and speed. Finally, I understood!

Then it was my turn, so I nervously glided out from the circle of people. Ready to test my new understanding, I skated my back crossovers to a step forward into an axel and then jumped off my left. As I turned, transferring my weight to the right, I felt an incredible sensation of flight and then sudden impact as my right foot hit the ground. I was centered. (I found myself wondering if this was how my dad felt when he was landing an airplane. No wonder he loved it.)

"Can you believe that?" a brunette on the sidelines grumbled. "It took me months to learn that move, and that kid nails it on the first try! That's not fair!"

"Yeah," the red-haired girl beside her grinned. "He's a natural."

"Let's see it again," the coach said. Again, I executed the jump, but this time I hit it off center. I slipped when my right foot hit the ground, and down I went.

"Do it again," he said.

I repeated the moves, and this time it worked. After crossing the threshold to this new and more intense level of skating, I knew that even more complicated jumps lay ahead. My passion was ignited, and the future looked better than ever.

My week at R.I.T. was so great that I called my folks and asked them if I could stay another week for my birthday. They said yes. This first summer laid the groundwork for the path that led me into the world of competitive skating. Not only did I learn new moves and dances, but I also became well-grounded in the basics, including the exacting task of school figures.

At the end of the second week, I was prepped and ready to take my first figures test. With so much importance placed on figures, it's understandable why my coach ordered me to practice them over and over. Because of the discipline required, my mom said that once I learned to focus on doing the figures, my school grades started improving. But all the focusing and practice in the world couldn't help me prepare for my test. I was only twelve years old and more nervous than I'd ever been. The formality of the situation didn't help, either.

Looking rigid and stern, the judges stood in a straight line on the ice. Both the men and women wore hats and long winter coats to ward off the ice-generated cold. We were required to skate up to them and perform our compulsory school figures, but the fifteen-minute exercise tested far more than just our skating skills.

At least when you're first, you get it over with quickly. The closer you are to the end of the line, the harder the wait. It's hard enough to take a test when nobody else can see what you're doing, but when you're performing in front of judges, family, and friends, it makes it that much harder when you mess up! At least, that's what my mind chewed on while I watched others ahead of me take their turns.

No matter how hard I tried to control it, I started to cry because I was so nervous. I sat on the bench, hunched over with my hands between my knees, and listened to myself mumbling, "This is way too hard. I can't do it. Maybe I don't have to do this."

"Are you ready, Scott?" My coach tapped me on the shoulder. I quickly wiped away my tears and then looked at my mom, who was sitting in the stands with the few remaining parents whose children were yet to perform. She nodded her head in a particular way that told me everything would be okay and I could do it.

"You're next," the coach informed me. There was no turning back: I was committed to go through with this.

Fear shot from my stomach to my throat and back again. Despite my wobbling knees, I pushed off with my right foot and then my left as I skated up to the line of judges. The rink's frigid air magnified the scraping sounds of my skates as they cut jagged lines into the ice. I could almost feel my mom holding her breath, like at the circus when the high-wire guy is about to perform a death-defying feat.

"You may begin," the head judge said, his pencil making a check with his right hand on the clipboard cradled inside his left arm.

And so I did. At some point during the test, my knees stopped shaking. Before I knew it, I was finished, so I returned to my spot before the judges.

"Very good," the head judge said. "Go take a seat. We'll bring the papers to you."

Another wait. I knew I'd done everything that I was supposed to, but I wasn't sure *how well* I'd done it. In my mind, I started reviewing my routine. I started second-guessing my performance, wondering if I could have done more or practiced more. I was frustrated because I couldn't go back and fix it.

After ten minutes of fretting, the head judge interrupted my misery by handing me the test papers. I passed. I passed! I passed! I looked at my mom and waved, the huge grin on my face telling it all.

"Congratulations," Coach Paikin said, patting me on the back. "You should be proud of yourself."

"Thanks," I said, flipping my skates into my bag. I did it! I couldn't believe that I really did it.

"This won't be your last time, you know."

I stopped. "What?"

"Scott, you've got an incredible future ahead of you."

"Uh, thanks," I replied, running toward my mother, who was making her way out of the stands. "Did you see me, Mom? How'd I do?"

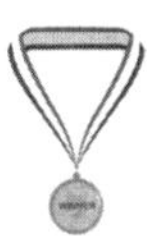

Back in Skaneateles, the summer was galloping to an end, so I filled the remaining days with my friends on the lake. One of the best parts of the summer was spent walking along the lake shore to my favorite "alone spot," a cave made with brush and shrubs. I lay down facing the lake, able to see the other side a mile away. I was perfectly hidden in my own little world. In this seclusion, I entertained deep thoughts about myself and my future. It was there that I realized I didn't want to be a pilot like my dad, a fireman, or a policeman. My thoughts embraced skating. As I gazed at the glistening water, my mind's voice said, *You're a good skater. Everyone says so, even the judges! If you put your mind to it, you could do something with this.* I liked going to this spot. Every time I went, I received reassurance and confirmation about my decision to continue my journey on the ice.

Even away from my hiding place, I couldn't quite get my mind off the sport. By October, signs started going up around town for hockey tryouts with the various youth leagues. That meant the rink would be opening soon, and I could hardly wait.

Unfortunately, we shared the rink with the hockey players. It was hard not to be distracted by helmeted and heavily padded guys impatiently waiting at the rink's edge for their turn. In most cases, being the only boy in the ice skating group brought unwelcome attention from the bystanders.

Ice time was precious, so we squeezed every last second out of our allotted time. As soon as the clock's sweep hand ticked to the top of the hour, the hockey jocks were on the ice, not giving us a chance to depart. Rudeness was inbred into these titans on ice from the beginning, so it was not unusual to be intentionally jostled, pushed, and shoved by the teens.

"Hey, Gregory, when are you going to stop playing with the girls?" Butch, the middle school bully, yelled from center rink. His cronies surrounded him, laughing and shoving. The first time Butch pulled that stunt, I started for center rink to punch him out.

"Don't, Scott." Coach Paikin placed a restraining hand on my shoulder. "It's not worth it."

I hesitated a moment. Five against one was not in my favor. Besides, they had sticks, but not as big as the one my mom would use if I started a fight for any reason.

"Yeah," I grumbled. "You're right."

My hope that Butch would keep our differences at the rink were quickly dashed. He came to school the next day, looking for me.

My friend Tommy and I were standing at our lockers between classes when Butch and the other hockey jocks showed up. Butch resembled a junior Norse god, minus the beard. His long, stringy blond hair was not one of his best features.

"Gregory, so you want to skate with the girls, huh?" Then he turned to his buddy. "I'd say he looks like a girl-skater, wouldn't you?"

The guys started punching each other while laughing. Before I could respond, they all walked away.

"You're the one who looks like a girl with your long hair and all," I muttered as I pulled my locker open.

Fortunately, they didn't hear me because of all the noise they were making.

"What was that all about?" Tommy asked while slamming his locker door shut.

"Hockey players think they're so tough," I replied.

The warning bell rang before Tommy could respond. English class beckoned.

With the exception of Butch's harassment, 1973 was a good year. Coach Paikin was pleased with my progress on the ice, and my parents were happy with my rapidly improving grades. They rewarded me with a full summer at R.I.T.

During my first year, I met a few guys, but that wasn't really long enough to get to know anybody. The second year was a different story. That was my summer with Bill Tillman from Philadelphia. We wandered around the campus and took everything in. In the process, we managed to get into mischief as only thirteen-year-olds can.

I also met a lot of girls at summer camp because the ratio was about thirty girls for every one guy. I was kind of shy when it came to girls, but ice dancing served as a great equalizer.

There weren't a whole lot of guys around, so we'd buddy up with some of the older girls. I felt like I was a high-level skater because I was hanging out with high-level skaters. It's like that old saying, "If you want to fly like an eagle, don't hang around the turkeys."

I would spend my free time at the rink, mimicking the advanced dancers. There was always a group of us that would hang out and watch the electronic board on the wall above the music room. When "Rumba" flickered on the board lighting up the letters for the next dance, we watched older skaters practice.

Then our little group would gather at the north end of the rink and practice along with the more advanced skaters. Laughing at our own foolish attempts to perform these advanced techniques, we would do our best and then dutifully wait for the next song to begin. No one seemed to mind because it was summer camp, after all.

My ice dancing coach was Dale Lynn. She paired me with Michelle Cerami during one of our first lessons, and we managed to stay together throughout the camp. Michelle had a bob haircut, brown hair, and blue eyes. Although she was smaller than I, we looked very much alike. In fact, we could have passed for brother and sister.

During the camp, we worked so well together that our parents and coaches decided we should compete together after the summer. There was only one problem: Michelle lived in Erie, Pennsylvania, more than two hundred and fifty miles away from me. But I was serious about my skating, so I wanted to make this happen.

To fit our schedules, we settled on weekend practice sessions together. Since my dad was an airline pilot, I could fly for free. So, on Saturday afternoons, I flew from Rochester to Pittsburgh and then picked up a connecting flight to Erie. Since we could only get late-night rink times, I would take a nap after I got there, and then we'd skate all night. I flew back home on Sunday and was back at school, with my homework done, on Monday.

Being given the responsibility to fly alone and back so often was something kids my age rarely had a chance to do, but I was a unique hybrid. I was still a kid who liked to do kid things, yet I was also an ice skater—an athlete who wanted to pursue his sport and strive for excellence. I had taken that first tentative step toward a commitment to persevere which is the basis of a champion mindset.

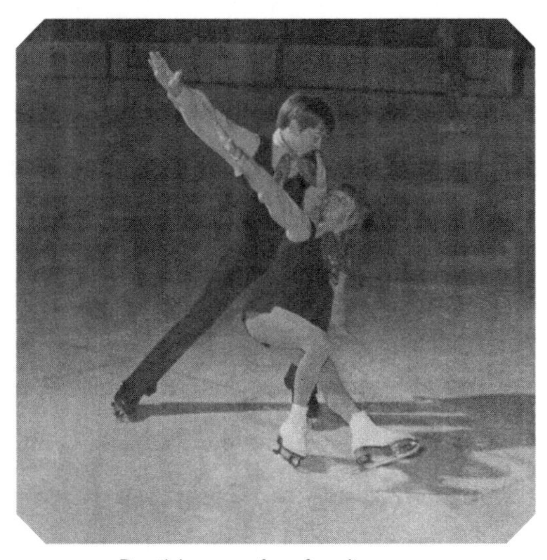

Practicing one of our favorite moves
with Michelle Cerami of Erie, PA.

Chapter 4

Greater Expectations

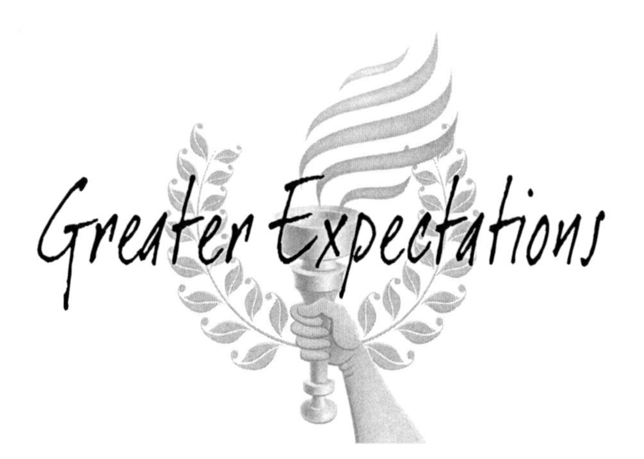

To successfully navigate the road to the top, athletes must engage in discipline, maintain focus, embrace commitment, and willingly step into the unknown. My early years on the lake, group and private lessons, and R.I.T. all played a part in setting me on a course that would take me deeper into the world of competitive figure skating.

While R.I.T. opened the door to an expanded skating experience, it was my mom and dad who kept the door open. Since Dad was away a lot, Mom was the one who conferred with my coaches and made sure I got the best practice times.

After we realized a change of coaches was needed, my parents made one of their most strategic moves ever. Richard Callahan, a seasoned national skater and now coach, was living and teaching in Rochester. Average in height, red-haired, and in his early thirties, Richard was an outstanding skater who was at R.I.T. during my second summer at the training camp. He would drive to Syracuse twice a week to teach at the state fairgrounds rink.

After just coming off the Ice Capades circuit, Richard skated and demonstrated a lot of the moves he expected me to achieve, such as a double Lutz or a double Axel. His level of expertise gave me something to aspire to. While I wasn't at that level then, I knew it was within reach, and Richard did too. His confidence in my potential inspired me to meet or exceed his expectations.

Richard had taken his skills further up on the skating scene. Placing fifth at the U. S. National Championships, he had already competed at a higher level than my first coach. Richard was able to build on the solid foundation that Michael had instilled in me by focusing on the technical and mental end of skating. His attention to detail brought me to a whole new level, preparing me for more intense skating competition. That preparation was tested when I competed in an open competition in Toronto, Canada, at the age of fourteen.

The rink was really cold, despite the fact that it was summer. There were four rinks under one roof, which was ideal since simultaneous events were in progress. Mine was rather small, and there wasn't much seating. You had to step way down (or so I thought because of my size) to get onto the ice.

As I waited for my turn to skate, I paced around in the crowded lobby adjacent to the rink. I stayed rather close to the doors that opened into the competition area so I wouldn't miss my cue. I felt a bit better when the skater ahead of me started his piece.

But as I watched him through the door's small window, he threw up. "Oh, no!" I whispered to no one in particular. "Oh, no, that didn't happen!" I murmured again as I turned away from my vantage point.

"What happened?" asked a blond boy about my age.

"That kid just got sick!"

"Wow!" he replied, "I've got to see that." I watched him barrel through the door. Shaking my head, I returned to the window, only to see the judges send the sick skater off the ice while rink maintenance shoveled up the mess. Ten minutes later, the boy returned to the hastily-cleaned ice and finished.

My knees started shaking as I struggled to control my fears. My turn came much too quickly, and I just didn't feel ready. I was so afraid because I was expecting the worst, and I lived up to these expectations. My mind went blank halfway through my program. I forgot everything, so I started skating around in circles. When I looked over at the board for Richard, he motioned for me to jump! I did a couple of double-toe loops until the music switched to more familiar areas. So I picked it up, got back into the program, and finished the routine. I learned then that you can't just quit in the middle of your program; you have to finish it, no matter what.

Maybe I was nervous because of what that boy before me did, or perhaps it was due to the lingering smell in the arena. I don't think I did very well that time, but it was one of those moments that taught me how to handle situations that may come up unexpectedly.

Presentation is of vital importance. For that first skating season with Richard, I wore a brown one-piece costume tastefully accented with a matching bow tie that I affectionately called "the monkey suit."

In August, two months before my first regional competition with Richard, he pulled me aside. "So, Scott, I want you to know and understand that you are an exceptional skater."

"Thank you," I said, a bit flustered. I wasn't used to receiving compliments, especially from Richard. I knew from my experience at R.I.T. that his praise wasn't easily earned.

"And exceptional skaters need exceptional skates," he continued as he handed me a worn pair of top-quality brown skates.

"What?" These were expensive skates. My parents were paying for my lessons and all other expenses, but skates like these certainly weren't in the budget.

"They were my skates in the Ice Capades."

"Really?"

"They served me well through the years. Try them on. They'll give you an edge."

The pro skates were a little heavier than my original ones but well suited for my routine and outfit. This was proven in the North Atlantic Regional Championships at the Amherst Skating Club near Buffalo, New York, in October 1973, when I competed at the intermediate men's level.

Much to my surprise, I came in second in school figures, which was sixty percent of our score. This gave my confidence level a real boost for the remainder of the competition.

Now, my Dad has always been a go-getter. After I finished skating my freestyle program, which followed the next day, Dad hurried up to the top of the bleachers and into the hallway, making sure he was among the first to see the judges' posted scores. Other family members were seconds behind, but he maintained his position at the front of the line. Not a word was spoken as the anxious adults milled around the board. About ten minutes after the event was over, a short, white-haired man who seemed filled with self-importance worked his way through the crowd and tacked a paper to the bulletin board.

While I was changing clothes, the drama unfolded upstairs. After Dad finished reading the newly posted scores, he sprinted to the steps leading to the lobby. I had just stepped out of the locker room when I saw him at the top of the final twelve metal steps leading away from the bleachers. He skipped from the landing, hitting every other step and over the final four, and positioned himself right in front of me! He grabbed my shoulders.

"You won!"

"What?" I couldn't believe him.

Dad was grinning from ear to ear, nodding his head up and down. "You won!"

I couldn't believe it. I had won Regionals, which meant that I would be competing at Sectionals, the next competition level. Only the top four in each category can go to Sectionals, and I was one of them! But the good news didn't stop there: Michelle and I won the Bronze dance competition.

We celebrated well that night. The next day, we were right back at work.

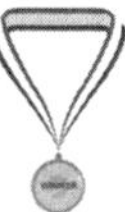

I learned from Richard that the greater the effort you put into your work, the better the results in the end. Part of that effort was getting to his lessons twice a week, and the other part was finding someplace to practice every day. That level of practice exceeded the available rink time in Skaneateles, so we gained ice time at rinks in Syracuse, Courtland, and Rochester.

Richard wasn't the first to recognize my potential. My parents actually saw the champion in me much earlier in the development process. While I enthusiastically embraced every new adventure, they cautioned me to use my time wisely. I heard their warnings but didn't fully understand until one day in the fall of 1973.

It was mid-morning on Saturday in Rochester. While waiting for my lesson, I focused on my freestyle moves. About fifteen minutes into the session, I noticed a friend of mine by the boards.

"Hey, Tony," I called as I skated toward him. "What do you think of Lucy? Do you think she's cute?"

Before he could answer, I heard my mom call me from the opposite end of the rink.

"Scott, could I see you for a moment, please?" Her arms were folded in front of her, with a sweater draped over them. She had the look that meant she was all business.

"Be right back," I called over my shoulder while pushing off the boards and heading toward my mother.

"Scott, how badly do you want this?"

Her question threw me. "What?"

"If you want this, don't waste your time on the ice. If you really want this, we're more than willing to pay for it; but if you fool around and talk, we're taking it away."

"Mom," I stumbled for words. "I was just, just—" but she stopped me mid-sentence.

"This is not a social event. Don't waste your ice time. It's too hard to come by. You can talk after your session."

Then she turned and walked away. "I'll see you later," I called to Tony as I skated back to center rink. While practicing my jumps and spins, I thought about what my mother just said, and I realized she was right. Her words became an anchor for me. For the first time, I knew that if I wanted to skate, I needed to take it seriously—practice time included.

When you're doing something you love that gives you satisfaction and builds you up while you strive for excellence, sacrifices become part of the process. Some might say that I sacrificed part of my childhood to pursue my goal, but that's just not so. Skating made my childhood better because it helped me grow and prove that I could be trusted.

One evening, my dad came home with a big grin on his face.

"Did you get it?" Mom asked as he strolled through the door.

"Yep," he said, looking quite pleased with himself.

"Get what?" I asked, peering over the open refrigerator door.

"What will it cost?" Mom said.

"Nothin'," he replied.

I shut the refrigerator door quietly.

"What costs nothing?"

"You need to get to bed early tonight, Scott," Dad said as he pulled his hand out of his pocket and showed me what rested in his palm—a plain, old key.

"Why?" I hesitated. "What's that?"

"You, my son, will have access to the Skaneateles Skating Rink so you can practice before school starts."

"What?" I couldn't believe it. I started jumping up and down in the kitchen as I grabbed the key from his hand.

Though I did go to bed an hour earlier, I found it hard to go to sleep that night. Only Dad could have pulled this off, since he knew all the town's movers and shakers. I wondered what he told them about me. What were their expectations? The questions rolled over in my mind until I finally drifted off.

"Come on, Scott. It's time to get up!"

My dad's voice ripped me from a sound sleep.

"Coming!" I moaned and groaned as I turned over and stretched. I lifted my head from the pillow and saw my green skate bag packed and ready to go.

"Now, Scott."

"I'm coming, Dad." The hands on my bedside clock told me it was 5 a.m. Looking out the bedroom window, I noticed that darkness still prevailed because dawn was a good ninety minutes away.

Moments later I was up, dressed, and hauling my green bag downstairs.

"Your toast is ready. Let's go," Dad said, heading out the back door to warm up our green Thunderbird.

Steam wafted off my cinnamon toast with icing as I juggled it with my overloaded skate bag. Nudging the door open, I navigated the short hallway and entered the garage, where I joined Dad. Once in the car, we were on our way to the rink, a good five-minute drive from our house.

"Got both sets of skates?" Dad asked, rehearsing the checklist that Mom gave him the night before.

"Yeah," I replied, my mouth full of chewy cinnamon toast. "Feestle and fibbers."

"What? Scott, don't try to talk with your mouth full. I can't understand a word."

"Freestyles and figures," I repeated, with a gulp. "I have both sets of skates and all my gear."

"And the key?"

"Yep, right here," I patted my chest.

"Don't lose it," he said as we pulled up to the rink.

"I won't." I got out of the car, grabbed my gear and headed toward the padlocked gate.

"I'll be back at 7:30 to take you to school."

"See ya!"

Alone at last. I pulled off my mittens, unshackled the gate, gained easy access, pulled my skate bag through, and then locked the gate up again. I groped my way to the Zamboni room and turned on the fluorescent lights. During the ten minutes it took for the lights to come on, I stayed in this room where compressors ran constantly, making the room warmer. After putting on my skates, hat, and gloves, I waited for the lights to come on in the rink. When the blue-tinged light filtered through the window of the exit door, I pushed the door open to enter the rink.

The familiar hum of the fluorescent lights greeted me, accentuating the rink's emptiness. Exterior canvas walls served as a wind-break of sorts. Before long, the sun would start peeking in the rink.

Gauging my time by the position of the sun, I switched skates about halfway through my practice session. I dedicated the first half to school figures and the last half to freestyle skating. Sometimes the maintenance workers would arrive before I finished. Their friendly greetings reconnected me to humanity, indicating that it was time to remove my skates and return to the outer world.

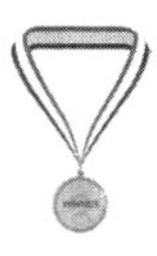

Skating like this in the early morning solitude was one of my favorite things to do. Every day it felt new and refreshing. This early-morning exercise was more about competing with myself than with other people, and I became more proficient and confident on the ice. It filled a deep need—a hunger to absorb everything that involved skating.

Early mornings at the Skaneateles rink were the best. I wish I could have had these private morning sessions all the time, but they were limited to the times when Dad was home and not flying for the airline. That was still okay with me because two or three times a week were a lot more than the other kids got. Besides, I had the key!

The early 1970s was definitely a time of infinite possibilities, especially in light of America's success with the Apollo space program. In 1969, Neil Armstrong became the first man to walk on the moon. In January 1971, the astronauts played golf there, and in 1972, NASA achieved its first successful night launch. It seemed like there was always one mission after another being launched.

One Friday afternoon, Mom picked me up after school to take me to Rochester to skate. Since it was Friday, I wasn't really interested in doing my homework. Instead, I listened to a talk radio station that was recapping the lunar expeditions.

"Mom?" I said, as the announcer summed up the leadership of the U. S. in the space race.

"What?" Mom's eyes were focused on the road ahead.

"We can achieve the impossible, can't we?" I was feeling awestruck by the magnitude of our country's achievements.

"What do you mean?" She obviously had something else on her mind.

"People used to think that putting a man on the moon was impossible, but now it's not. If we can do that, we can do just about anything!" I felt an undefined sense of enthusiasm and excitement welling up within me.

"I suppose so," she said.

As Mom focused on driving, my own thoughts began to embrace the possibility of doing more. If we could achieve space travel, what could I accomplish as a skater? Then I realized that there was no reason I couldn't achieve the impossible on the ice. My mind's eye captured a moment in the distant future, a glimpse of being a champion—the best.

I can do this, my mind's voice whispered. It wasn't an impossible dream. Lost in my thoughts, I was surprised at how quickly we arrived at the rink. I felt more highly motivated than ever before to fulfill my dream.

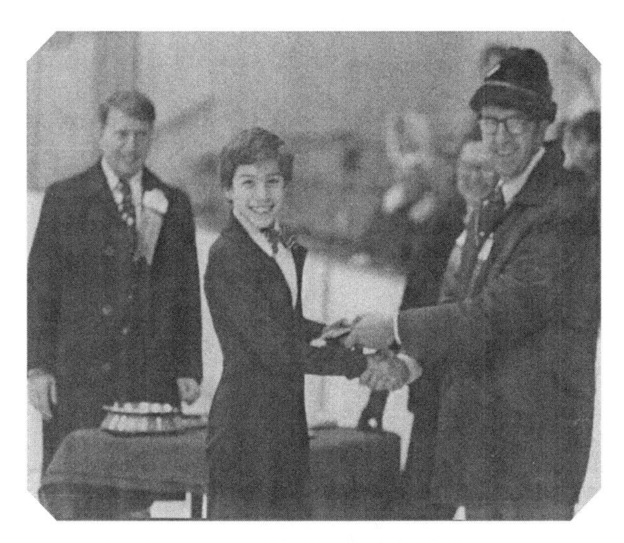

Receiving my award for Intermediate Men's Level
at North Atlantic Regional Championships.

Chapter 5

Discouraged, Never!

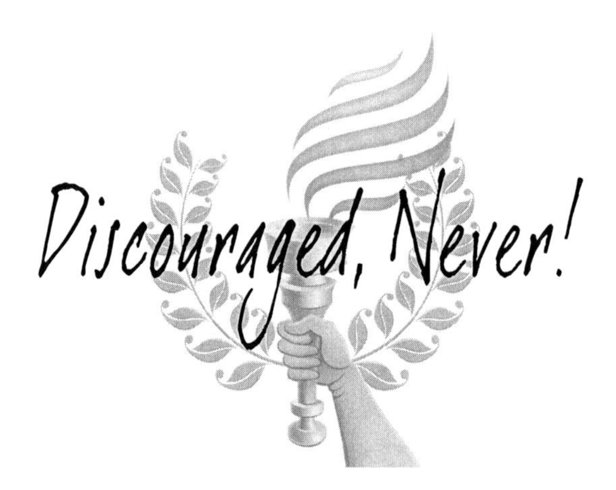

Working with Richard involved more practices and competitions. I tested and went up levels after successfully mastering new jumps, spins, and routines. Skating at each higher level meant an event with new and different pressures.

I needed to prove to myself that I could translate what I did in practice to excellent programs in front of the judges and audiences. Little did I know that my next decision would change everything.

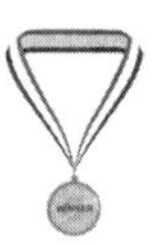

I had just turned fifteen when Richard called me into his office. I knew that he saw my potential and figured I could go further, with the right training and opportunities.

I sat down and dropped my skating bag onto the floor by my chair.

"You skated great today."

"Thanks," I said.

Richard cleared his throat, leaned back in his chair, and hesitated.

I sat quietly, wondering why he was stalling.

"Scott, I'm teaching in Philadelphia next month and will move there as soon as my wife and I can find a place."

"What!" I couldn't believe what I was hearing.

"And I want you to continue your skating and training with me in Philly. You can stay at our house."

My mind was groping to comprehend what he said. At first, I was devastated to think that my progress would stop, then elated that it wouldn't. But then, a harsh reality filled my thoughts. Training with Richard in Philadelphia meant that I would have to give up everything for my skating. I would have to give up my school friends, my mom and dad, my brother and sister, and the lake. I would have to leave everything behind that was familiar to me.

"But what about my p-parents?" I stuttered, my voice sounding more like a wounded frog than a person.

"I've already talked to your mom. If you want to continue your training with me, she said they would support the move."

I couldn't believe it. I was happy and sad at the same time. What did they think about my desire to leave them? Would they think that I didn't care about them anymore? I found out that night.

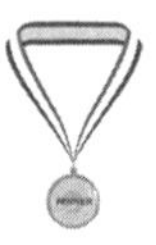

"Well," Mom said after we'd cleared the dishes and headed for the living room. "I understand Richard made you an offer . . ."

A nice warm fire cut the Indian summer chill. We all adjourned to our favorite seats. I preferred sitting on the couch facing the window because I loved looking out at the lake. Sunset was one of my favorite times, with its warm, purple-orange glow reflecting on the water below.

"What kind of offer?" Dad looked up, skeptical. "Did he find you a sponsor or something?" He reached to his left to turn off the television.

"No." I looked at my family, one by one. "Richard wants me to move to Philadelphia with him and his family."

"Next summer?" asked my sister, who looked a little bored.

"After Richard gets settled in. It should be in a few months," I corrected her.

"But what about school?" she screeched. She looked more upset than I thought she would be. After all, I was the pain-in-the-neck baby brother who was always getting in the way, wasn't I?

"I'll start here and then transfer to a school in Philadelphia." It was pretty clear to me, so what was *her* problem?

"Yeah?" She sounded even more defensive. Maybe I wasn't so hard to be around after all.

"If you guys say it's all right."

Then they all started talking at the same time. I kind of lost track of the arguments until Mom's voice calmed the cacophony.

"Then, it's settled. We all agree that Scott should have this chance."

"But—" Mom's look immediately silenced Heather's objections.

I was scared. As tough as early-morning departures, keeping my grades up, and practicing endless hours had seemed, moving away from everything I knew would be the hardest thing yet. Did I want it badly enough for a boy of fifteen?

Yes, I did. Every decision I had made to this point supported my sport. They weren't decisions considered normal for a guy living in a hockey town. Summers were the hardest, especially living where we did. While my friends were playing on the lake, I was always out of town, practicing my skating on a cold ice rink.

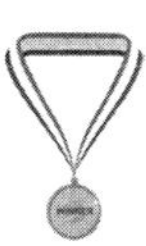

But there are times in life when a path appears before us. We have to choose which way to go. Making major life decisions is not just something that falls lightly on us; instead, it's a huge intersection in the road. Okay, which way should I go? I could either quit, stay home in Skaneateles and find a new coach, or take a faith-step into the unknown. I chose the faith-step.

I've always believed that things happen for a reason. God has a plan, and He gives us these decisions to make. Once made, we must live with them. I knew I was ready.

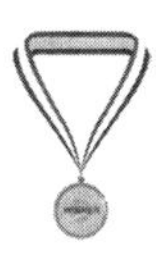

The next month, Richard assumed the position of head coach for the Philadelphia Skating Club and Humane Society, which dates back to 1849. Before I could join him, however, I had to be accepted into this prestigious organization.

It was during the fall of 1974, a few months after Richard's announcement. He had found a home, so it was time to initiate my move. The week before, we had received notice that the board would meet with my parents and me, so we had to drive from Skaneateles to Ardmore, almost two hundred and fifty miles away.

"Scott! Hurry up. We've got to leave."

"What's the hurry, Dad? I thought you said it would take five hours! It's only three o'clock in the morning."

"We've got weather. Now, get your stuff, and let's get moving!"

Dad was right. Our five-hour drive took more than eight during one of the worst ice storms in the region's history. With its rolling hills and sharp turns, Route 41, the back road along the lake, was more like a bobsled course. We breathed easier once we got to the Pennsylvania turnpike where snowplows diligently cleared the way for the heavily traveled road, so we could move a bit faster.

When we arrived at the skating club, we met the interviewers. One was scary looking, in a Count Dracula sort of way. He was tall with hairy eyebrows that stuck out and had hair coming out of his nose and ears.

"Mr. Gregory!"

I wondered if he could see his reflection in a mirror.

"Yes, sir." Even though their new head coach's sponsorship carried a lot of weight, I still needed to make a good impression.

"We understand that you want to become a member of our skating club. This is not an application we take lightly. Why do you want to join us?"

His voice resonated deep within me. *I want to come because my coach said I* had *to. But I can't tell them that. What should I say?*

I cleared my throat. "Because I want to keep getting better."

"Better than whom?"

"Better than me, better than I am now."

He leaned over and whispered to the lady sitting next to him. She nodded solemnly and wrote something on the paper in front of her. This made me even more nervous than Dad's battling two hundred and fifty miles of icy roads and almost zero visibility to get there.

"And what do you hope to achieve while you're here?"

How do I know what I want to achieve? I'm a kid who's never been away from home. I want to skate. I feel like I'll die if I don't skate!

"Well, sir." I looked around the room. Pictures of famous skaters lined the walls, along with shadow boxes filled with trophies, flags, and ribbons.

Then I remembered Richard telling me about the club's mantra—good conductivity, good sportsmanship, and participation in the club.

"Well, sir, I um . . ."

Good conductivity, good sportsmanship, and participation in the club.

"I want to learn to express good conductivity, good sportsmanship, and to participate . . ."

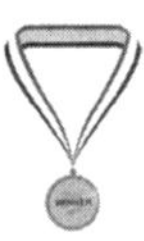

"Yes, very good." He was obviously satisfied. "Did you bring your skates?"

"Yes, sir."

"We'll see you on the ice in fifteen minutes."

Three weeks later, I received my acceptance letter from the Philadelphia Skating Club and Humane Society. My next priority focused on finding a high school that worked best with my training schedule. A private Catholic school, Archbishop Carroll High School near Villanova, met with everyone's approval. Not only did they have high academic achievement records, but they also offered me a flexible schedule to accommodate my skating, as well as acceptance of my training as credit for gym class. That meant I could come in later in the morning and leave school earlier in the day.

After I moved to Philadelphia, my life took on a new rhythm and pattern. School and skating consumed all my time. I would skate in the morning from 5:30 to 7:30, go to school, then *bam*, right back to the rink from 2:30 until 6:30. I'd go home, have dinner, and do homework. There was no time to socialize because skating, homework, and sleep took up my entire day.

Barely used to this new routine, much less preparing for the South Atlantic Regionals in Washington D. C., the event rolled around way too soon. In spite of Richard's reassurances, my confidence level was shot. I tried to intellectualize my fear. If reasoned that if I could identify it, I could conquer it: *my first competition away from the security of my childhood home; fear of failure while pursing my untested dream.* Now for the conquering part. All too soon, my name boomed through the loudspeaker. Muddle-minded and doubt-riddled, I stepped out on the ice and posed, waiting for the music to begin.

I've got to remember the routine. I can do this. I know I can. I silently repeated these thoughts when the music started.

I did well through the first ninety seconds, but as I finished one of my spins, I got disoriented. My mind went blank, and panic set in as I started skating in circles. It was Toronto all over again. I looked toward Richard, who was trying to discreetly signal my next move. Suddenly, the familiar music nudged me back to the routine that I had rehearsed daily since I moved to Philadelphia. Finally, the agony was over, and I skated off the ice. There was no point in wanting to know my placement because I knew that I had tanked.

"You'll do better next time," Richard said, patting me on the shoulder as I slumped onto the bench.

"Yeah, if there will be a next time," I groused.

Richard arched his eyebrow but chose not to say anything.

Mom and Dad were waiting for me outside the changing room after the program finished.

"Better luck next time," Dad said before I could utter a word.

"I want to come home," I said, humiliated by my failure.

"Not today," he said before Mom could reply. "You have a commitment to fulfill before you pack it in. Now, let's go get some dinner."

While we ate at a nearby restaurant, my parents talked about everything but my failure. Unusually quiet, I didn't eat much. All I wanted to do was hide under a rock.

Richard let me rest the next day, but on Monday morning he had me back on the ice at 5:30.

"You have some new jumps I want you to work on," Richard said.

"Okay," I replied, still stinging from the weekend's events.

"It's time for you to work on your double axel and triple-toe loop."

I felt half-hearted making the attempts, but these new incentives forced me to focus on the moves and kept me from dwelling on my failure.

After supper two days later, Richard handed me a letter from my dad. I went upstairs to my bedroom to read it in private. The letter was dated December 8, 1974:

Scott, my son,

Today my heart is heavy. Oh, how I wish I could be jubilant. It somehow was not the wish of our Supreme Father to grant you the chance to stand in the winner's circle. We all know that you have the ability, the desire, and the guidance.

Discouraged, never! Your mother can recall these words from her college days. I think of them often in these trying times. Many are the occasions when everything seems to go against us. This is the time for our inner soul to come forth and allow us the courage to try even harder.

Set yourself a goal. Make it a long way off, a goal that is almost unattainable. Through the years, you will find that the pathway to your goal has many pitfalls. This weekend surely is an example. You can, I know, find the strength to continue.

Some historians may have said it in different terms, but let me say, "Work diligently, persevere, and thou shalt conquer."

Instill your confidence, and you shall not fail.

Your admiring father,
Dad

I set the letter aside and fought back tears. All the frustration welled up within me, yearning for release. I felt like I was five years old, in my father's arms after a big fight with my older siblings; but I knew it would be all right because Dad was there, holding me. His letter made it better. Little did I know that this letter would become a cornerstone to the foundation of my future.

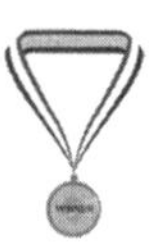

My first year away made me appreciate my family and home in Skaneateles even more. But I was happy, doing what I wanted to do most—skate. I made it through the year, competing heavily in the fall and mastering new skills in the winter.

However, this idyllic life was destined to be short-lived. As an athlete, I had experienced pain before. All athletes go through pain. In most cases, they just work through it if they have the right attitude. It's all part of running the race.

So I ignored it, even when the pain continued to increase. I took my dance and free-skating tests and kept on moving up levels . . . until I noticed a different kind of pain in my back and problems with my right knee. When I skated on the ice, I felt weak. This frustrated me because I couldn't put all my effort in the jumps. The more I jumped, the greater my pain. I was sore, unable to give the sport my full energy. It was like limping on a bad leg and favoring the pain.

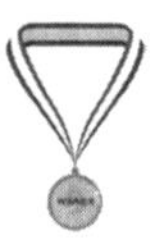

The doctors couldn't figure out what was going on, so they labeled it "growing pains" and told me to rest. That meant taking two weeks off from the ice, no option.

This was my first sports injury. Forced to stay off the ice with only homework and music to fill my days, my frustration level soared, and I felt defeated. Lying on my bed one afternoon, silent tears pooled in the corners of my eyes. "I'm Not in Love," by 10CC, played on the radio. My headsets kept the music personal, intimate, and just for me. When the lyrics "Big boys don't cry" enveloped me, that's all I could do. This was the first time I was so upset that I cried. I wasn't allowed to skate due to the injury that I didn't even know how I got! I hadn't bargained for this.

It's hard to be tough when you're hurting, but the song's message struck a chord deep within my soul. Some things are worth crying over, but others you just have to tough out. This was one of them, a message that I needed to remember—one that would help prepare me for bigger obstacles later on.

Staying off the ice for two weeks didn't do much to remove the pain in my back and knee. The pain was stealing my joy. A popular saying of the day was, "No pain, no gain." When I felt the pain, I didn't want to be a baby about it, but there was a limit to where I could push myself as a skater and an athlete. I learned too late how far I could push my body without breaking it.

If you have a drive when you're young and committed, and you want to be really good, you push through that stuff. You must be sensitive to hear what your body is saying day after day, and then act upon it. But realizing what you should do and doing it are often two separate things.

To accomplish the easier moves that were once second-nature to me, I focused on getting past the pain, but I couldn't concentrate on improving my performance. These pain-laced hours on the ice drove all the fun out of my dream. Maybe skating wasn't such a good idea after all.

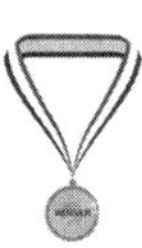

But how could I stop? I still loved the sport. My two weeks off the ice devastated me. My parents' faith in my commitment and talent bolstered me. My passion for the ice lived, despite the agony that overwhelmed me. I couldn't really comprehend leaving, so I let momentum carry me to the next level, the next event, and the next move.

I persevered and performed well enough to participate in summer skating camp near Buffalo. Since Toronto was less than two hours away, Richard signed me up for the Toronto Invitational Summer Competition.

When we arrived in Toronto, the weather was clear—a great day for competition. We were staying at Richard's sister's house, so we got plenty of rest the night before. His sister, a neat lady, said something that made a strong impression on me.

"Break a leg," she called after us as we walked down the steps toward the waiting car. She wasn't joining us at the arena.

That's corny, I thought as I climbed in after Richard and mentally prepared for the competition ahead.

Break a leg kept resonating in the back of my mind, but I laughed at the absurdity of the thought. After all, I'd never had any *real* trouble before. And this was the same competition where years earlier I had to skate after the boy who got sick. What could go wrong?

After gearing up, I entered the competition area. Canadian champion Toller Cranston, competing in the senior men's event, captivated thousands of fans in a rink on the north end of the building. It didn't seem like the same place where I competed years earlier.

As an intermediate skater, my events were on the south end of the arena. Bleachers filled with competitors' families and friends helped me tap into the excitement of the day.

Then it was my turn. The music started, and I began to skate. Everything was going well. I executed a perfect double flip and, moments later, picked into the ice for the Russian split jump. Before I could vault, however, I felt my leg buckle underneath me. I couldn't even get my foot off the ground. Pain exploded in my knee, and I collapsed. Seconds seemed like hours as I struggled to regain my footing. I looked up and saw Richard and a bunch of other people running out on the ice toward me.

Chapter 6

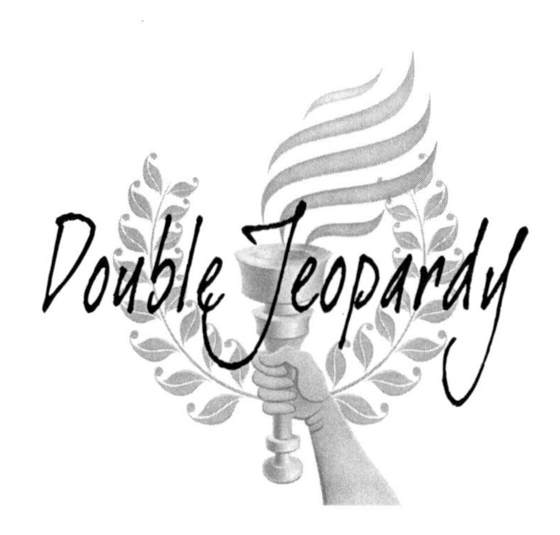

Double Jeopardy

Lying there on the ice, time slowed to a crawl, compounded by intense pain in my right leg. *What happened? Did my leg blow up? Where did this come from? This isn't fun!*

Hundreds of simultaneous thoughts swirled through my head, competing against the pain that surged through my knee. Minutes seemed like hours as my music still played, until the head referee realized that I was not going to get up again. A series of hand signals stopped the music and brought the medical staff onto the ice with a stretcher. They had to get me off the ice as quickly as possible so the competition could continue.

After the EMT's took me to a locker room, I sat up while the attending physician rolled up my pants leg. Instead of seeing a normal leg, I observed a sunken hole where my knee should have been. Extreme pain carried me into shock as I dropped back down onto the gurney. I later learned that picking in for the jump had split my kneecap in half.

The doctors at a nearby hospital patched me up as best they could and sent me home with instructions to see a specialist. That was the last time I ever skated at that rink in Toronto.

My mom wanted to make sure I had the right doctor, so she started searching. She found Dr. Joseph D. Godfrey, an orthopedic surgeon who was the team physician for the Buffalo Bills, a top NFL football team. It was clear that this injury was going to take me off the ice for a long time

The stress from my jumps had literally blown my kneecap apart. Surgery was the only option, so within a week, I was on Dr. Godfrey's operating table. Even though in real time a week wasn't long, it seemed like an eternity to me. I just wanted to get my knee fixed. I was only fifteen, so this wasn't supposed to be happening.

Time stood still on the operating table. One minute I was awake, and the next I was out. During the two-hour procedure, Dr. Godfrey made an incision in the skin over my kneecap, from one side to the other. Once the bone was laid bare, he pieced it together like a puzzle, inserted a screw to hold it in place, and then stitched me back up. Next came the cast, a full-leg plaster concoction that covered everything except my toes.

In the recovery room, the nurses kept turning me over to inject pain medication. I didn't feel so bad after I saw the guy next to me. He had been in a motorcycle accident and was totally immobilized. The nurses placed a mirror above him so he could see who was around.

After I remained in the hospital for a week, Dr. Godfrey sent me home to finish my recovery. Instead of a conquering hero, I returned to Skaneateles High School for my sophomore year like a broken eagle with its wings clipped. Rather than soaring on the ice, I was back in class on crutches.

The Vietnam War was still headline news. Horror stories of prisoners of war being tortured and put in small cages invaded the television screens. They were bent over and scrunched into a position where they couldn't stretch out. My immobility—not being allowed to move my leg, and keeping it straight for months—helped me sympathize with their plight.

Being in a cast is not fun at all; ask anyone who's suffered from a broken limb. If the aching doesn't do you in, the itchiness will drive you nuts and make you feel like screaming. Using a coat hanger, probably one of the worst things for scratching an itch, provides a little relief. But if you're not careful, you'll break the skin, and it will get infected. But that didn't stop me from scratching. I was lucky—stupid but lucky.

A few days after I got home from the hospital, Mom brought me a small book entitled *So Run Your Race: The Moral and Spiritual Odyssey of an Athlete*, by Patsy Neal.

"Read it," she said as she handed it to me.

I didn't have anything better to do, so I opened the sixty-three page book and started to read. I was quickly drawn into the free-verse style of Neal's book. As a three-time All-American women's basketball player and participant in international competitions, she was well-qualified to get into my head—and she did.

Through her words, I revisited my life, beginning as a child who yearned to skate on the ice like the big boys. As I grew, my play turned into a serious sport. With sport came the discipline to train and seek perfection. There was a great deal of work, pain, and practice involved, continuously embracing the perfect move to make my body do things most bodies don't or won't. That's where I was and what I had been doing until my injury.

Her book laid out a pattern, a road map of sorts. Little did I know that those sixty-three pages were prophetically revealing the road ahead. The prayer on page 37 especially spoke to my hurting heart: "I have seen You repair my bruised body, healing my sprains and torn muscles through the years of strain and struggle, without once taking away from the fun of jerking stops and painful moves. For even in the pain, You spoke to me of victory over the flesh . . ."

Then it hit me. I would recover, and I would skate again. I knew that I just *had* to skate. I went back to page 21. *I am a man now,* I thought. *I am strong. I am skilled. I can be a champion.*

I flipped to the front of the book to reread it from start to finish. I felt encouraged by the author's insight and her assurance that I wasn't alone in this battle. Yeah, I went to church with my parents when I was home, but this book opened the door to a spiritual understanding that would help prepare me for what lay ahead.

If I thought a few weeks off the ice was bad, taking months to recover was much worse. Instead of spending hours alone on the ice improving my skills, I was tossed into a social environment that gave me a new opportunity to develop school friends, something I didn't have time to do before.

Mobility was a bit of an issue, but I managed fairly well, despite my infirmity. If I couldn't be on the ice, at least I had the lake. One day, I borrowed my dad's 250-horsepower Century motorboat and went out on the water. I liked going out there because it was quiet, and I had time to think about what I wanted for the future. No matter how much I tried to shake it off, I couldn't get skating out of my system.

Drifting closer to the shore, I decided to cruise the lake's perimeter and found myself drawing closer to town. As I nosed toward the small pier, I saw a familiar face.

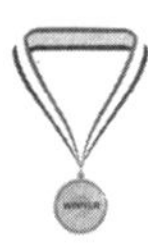

"Hey, Scott!" I heard Chuck Borschuk call my name as I was pulling into the dock in downtown Skaneateles. A taller, light-haired, muscular fellow was right behind him.

With the bow line in one hand, I started to use my crutch to leverage myself onto the wooden pier. Chuck's friend, who was built more like a wrestler, came running toward me, grabbed my arm, and hoisted me onto the dock. Before I could object, he took the bow line and secured it to the metal cleat on the dock.

"Nice boat," he said, looking over my shoulder.

"It's my dad's," I replied.

"Aren't you afraid of falling out of the boat with that cast on your leg?"

"Who is this guy?" I asked Chuck who was still standing on the pier.

"Don Matson," he said. "Don, this is Scott Gregory. You know, he's the figure skater I told you about," Chuck added, doing an ice-hockey version of a pirouette.

I just sighed and started to walk toward town.

"What happened to your leg?" Don asked, slowing down to walk beside me.

"Russian split," I replied, hobbling as fast as my cast would let me.

"Is that hard to do?" His question stopped me where I stood.

"What?"

"The Russian split. Is it hard to do?"

"I don't know," I said, continuing my walk. "My knee broke in half when I picked in for the jump, so for me at that moment, yeah. I guess it was pretty hard. Why?"

"I don't know. Just curious, I suppose."

"Do you skate?"

"A little," he replied. "Where did it happen?"

"In Toronto."

"Toronto? What were you doing there?"

I stopped suddenly. "I was in a skating competition."

"Whoa! That's pretty cool."

"It is?" His reaction surprised me. "I think so."

Unlike most of the male population at Skaneateles High School, Don didn't poke fun at me or my sport. After that, we became fast friends, a friendship that would continue for the rest of our lives.

When I finally got the cast off, I had to work doubly hard to get ready for the ice. That time of rebuilding was intense, painful, and frustrating. Prior to this, I had never done any off-ice conditioning; but now I needed to strengthen my leg, which had lost much of its muscle mass after being in a cast for two months.

The neat thing about exercise is that you can do it just about anywhere. My usual spot was at home on the stairs in the hallway that separates the kitchen from the television room. It had everything I needed, including a sturdy banister that held my weight when I was younger. I would slide down it when I thought Mom wasn't looking.

The exercise was called a step-up. I would hold onto the banister for balance as I repeatedly stepped up on one step and back down.

Right leg, step up, step back down.

"Scott!" Mom's voice threatened to derail my hundred-step count.

Right leg, step up, step back down.

"Tell your brother that dinner's almost ready."

Right leg, step up, step back down.

"Bee Gee! Mom says—"

"I'm on the phone, man," Bee Gee's voice countered from the TV room.

Right leg, step up, step back down, seventeen.

"Mom, Bee Gee says—"

Right leg, step up, step back down, twenty-two.

"Now, you boys hurry up! I don't want your dinner to get cold!"

Right leg, step up, step back down, thirty-one.

"Bee Gee, Mom says now!"

Right leg, step up, step back down, forty-six.

"All right, I'm coming!?" Bee Gee's voice right next to me startled me off step.

"Aw! I'm halfway there. I'll have to finish my flexes later."

I did a hundred step-ups, at least twice a day. I couldn't wait to get back on the ice. Much later, I learned that off-ice training like this was crucial for avoiding injury.

I continued to faithfully exercise until Dr. Godfrey finally cleared me to skate. With my wait over, I called Richard and told him I was coming back.

Chapter 7

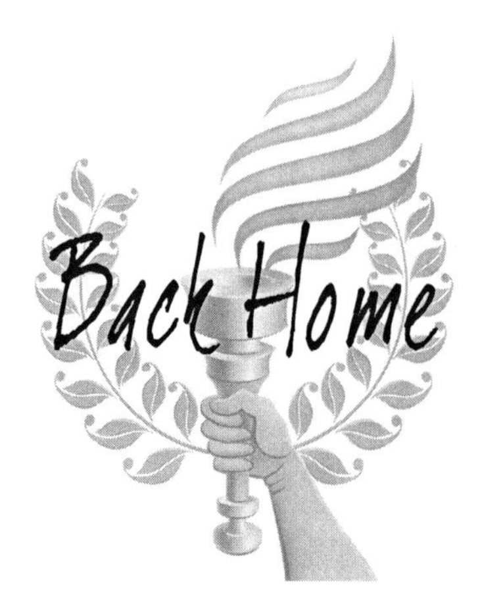

Back Home

While I was recuperating in Skaneateles, Richard accepted a coaching position in Buffalo, New York. When it was time to join him there, I focused on improving my skating. I was always among the first at the rink in the morning and gained as much practice time as I could. He had arranged for me to stay with the Hatchst family, who lived in a rural residential area in Buffalo.

I particularly enjoyed listening to Grandpa Hatchst's stories about his childhood and immigrating to the United States from Budapest. He was about my age when he worked as a mechanic on airplanes at the Buffalo Airport in the early 1920's. I normally found him in front of the television with a magnifying glass watching stock quotes.

The Hatchst's daughter, Lisa, was a senior at Amherst High School. Because she was a grade ahead of me and had her own friends, we rarely saw each other during the day.

Mrs. Hatchst accepted me as someone focused and dedicated to my sport. She pretty much expected me to do my own thing and stay out of trouble. She figured I was responsible enough to get myself to school, and she was right. I could take care of myself, except at mealtimes, which was all right because she was such a great cook.

A few days after I moved in, I met a guy in one of my classes at school named Jorge Rodriguez. Coincidentally, he was staying with an American family just ten doors down the street from where I was living.

Jorge was a year older than I. Originally from Costa Rica, he was visiting the United States to improve his language skills. Rather short and boxy with dark brown eyes so deep that they almost looked black, Jorge's features and engaging accent set him apart from the typical northern New Yorker.

We soon became fast friends, even though Jorge wasn't a skater. Always upbeat, he found the sport of ice skating intriguing. When we had some leisure time, we listened to music together, especially Santana, one of our favorite groups. Otherwise, my spare time was spent at the rink.

Richard suggested that I train for both singles and possibly dance competitions. He said that ice dancing would help further my career. After just coming off my injury, dancing would not be as challenging for my knee. So he paired me with a local skater, Patty Edict. Our goals were to work at developing a partnership and then see how far we could get on the competition scene.

My free-skating wasn't progressing as quickly as I would have liked. When the doctor said I was well, I figured that I was *totally* well and could rush right back into things. In my mind, I was invincible, and nothing else could go wrong. I wanted to do all the things I could do before my injury, like performing jumps again. But Richard kept saying that I wasn't ready.

Working with my new partner helped. I employed various techniques and learned new dances with Patty. Richard promised to increase my training schedule after the holidays. Late November came quickly, and the Thanksgiving break opened the door for a short visit home.

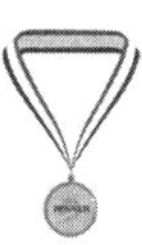

Shortly after I arrived in Skaneateles, Don Matson called and asked me to join him at the rink the next morning.

I was up bright and early the next day when I ran into my mother in the kitchen. She was in the middle of packing the car with her ski stuff.

"Where you going?"

"To Song Mountain for the day to do some skiing. Do you want to come?"

Snow-skiing was Mom's second passion, and Song Mountain was only forty minutes away.

"Nah. Don's coming over. We're going to the rink."

"I thought you got enough of skating in Buffalo," she laughed.

"I can never get enough of skating."

"Be careful, honey. Don't do anything stupid."

"Yeah, yeah, I won't. See you tonight."

I was feeling good, strong, invincible—and anxious. I couldn't handle too many days away from my skating. When Don finally showed up, I was more than ready.

I jumped in his turquoise van, and we drove to the rink. It was a sunny, snowy day—sunny one minute and snowing the next. Like so many mornings before, the rink was cold but inviting.

Lacing up my left boot first and then my right, I got that familiar, excited feeling that comes whenever I'm getting ready to skate. It's my routine. Changing it would be next to *impossible.* Left foot first; then right foot. It just feels right.

Even though it was a public session, the rink was almost empty.

"It seems weird not meeting you at lunch and after classes," Don said, as he sat beside me.

"It's different," I replied, eager to start skating for fun.

"What's it like?"

"I practice in the morning before I go to school, go to the rink after classes are over, and work until dinner time. Then I go home, eat, and do homework."

"No time for fun, eh?" he laughed, punching my arm.

"Skating is fun," I replied, jumping up and getting on the ice before he even had a chance to finish lacing.

I started going through my moves while Don circled the edge of the rink like a polar bear. I could tell he was impressed, because each move I executed was a bit more complicated than the last. Then I was ready for my one of my favorite moves, the most impressive in my arsenal at the moment. Don was rounding a corner, so his back was to me.

"Hey, Don," I called out, circling around to set up my jump. Anticipation of the thrill and admiration in his eyes filled me. "Watch this!"

I was so engaged in the moment that I failed to notice a slight weakness in my knee. My toe-pick snagged the ice as I prepared for my Russian split. As the momentum built and I heaved my legs up for the split, I felt it. My right leg stayed put, carrying all the weight and pressure of my body. Pain erupted from my knee, emanating outwards. Then, *bam*! Down I went.

What? Not again? It can't be happening again!

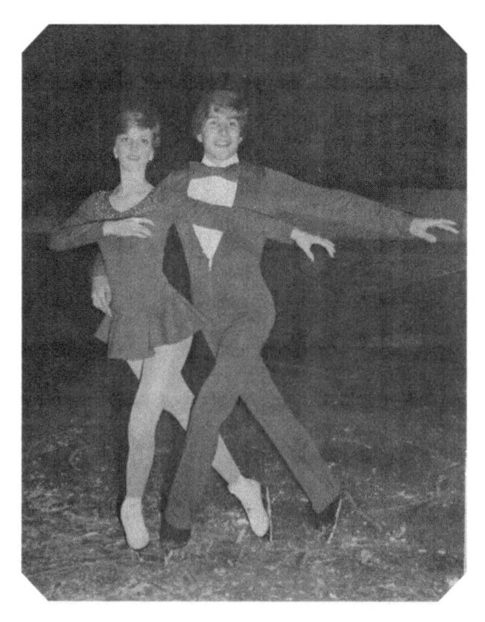

Patty Edict and I skated together only a couple months due to my second injury.

Chapter 8

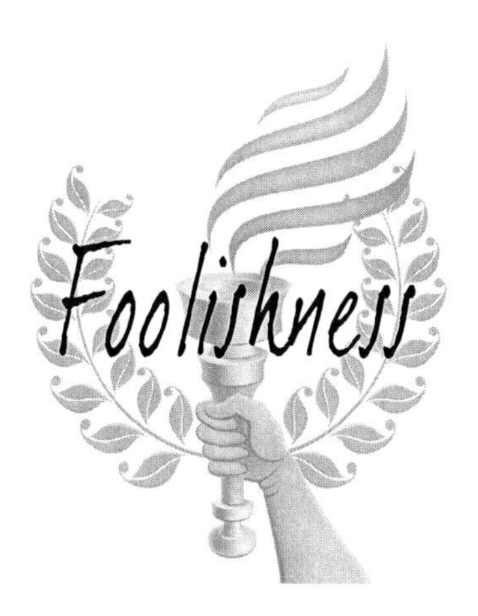

Feelings of stupidity for trying the Russian split had just cost me my skating career. My mother was right to warn me not to do something *foolish.* Sitting there with both legs stretched out in front of me, my back straight, and my fists pounding the ice revealed just how stupid I felt.

"I did it again!" I reached over and pulled my pant leg up. The skin over my kneecap was soupier than before. It looked worse than the first time it was broken.

That's it. I'm done. I can't recover from another year off this ice. It might as well be forever. My mind was in a muddle. I was so mad that I couldn't talk, as I tried to hold back tears of pain and thoughts of never skating again.

Don tried to help me off the ice, but he couldn't move me without causing more pain. So he went to the office and phoned my mom while a rink guard called an ambulance, which arrived rather quickly. At least

I wasn't in a major public venue like the last time. Still, I didn't like the helplessness I felt as they loaded me onto the gurney and strapped me in.

I can't believe this. This can't be happening! Will I be able to start all over? It's not fair. It's not fair!

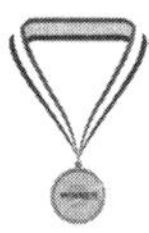

Don rode with me in the ambulance that took me to the hospital in Auburn, where my worst fears were confirmed. The doctors put my leg in an immobilizer until I could see Dr. Godfrey.

When Mom came in, she looked ashen, older than she appeared that morning. I could see my fear reflected in her face.

"I did it again, Mom," I said.

"I knew you'd been hurt. When I heard the page, I was on my way up the slope."

"It's not fair, Mom. Why should this be happening to me?"

"Everything happens for a reason. You're strong. Let's see what the doctors have to say and focus on getting you back on your feet."

That's not what I wanted to hear. I wanted to be back in Buffalo, now. I got my wish, but not the way I expected.

The doctors sent me home for a day to prepare for surgery. Mom made arrangements to admit me to the hospital in Buffalo and drove me up the next day. When Dr. Godfrey examined my knee, he just shook his head.

"Well, Scott, it looks like you did it again," he said after removing the immobilizer.

"Tell me about it," I grumbled.

"I'll do what I can, but it doesn't look like you'll ever be able to skate again."

A big lump formed in my throat as he pulled my mom aside and started talking to her.

Later that afternoon, we learned that my surgery was scheduled for the next day. This time he took bone marrow from my hip and grafted it into each side of the kneecap. Then he reconnected the two broken pieces with a long titanium screw. The screw was prominent enough that, when x-rayed, the head on one side of my knee and the sharp tip slightly protruding on the other could be clearly seen. This screw was designed to remain in my knee where the first one was removed after eight months. Dr. Godfrey said the repair would be stronger this time, but he still warned me not to skate.

Mom stayed at Richard's house while I was in the hospital. It was the easiest way to keep him in the loop and shortened the commute during my week in bed.

Depression seemed to be my constant companion during my hospital stay. That's when a surprise visitor changed the entire tone of my recovery.

"Scott? Are you awake?"

Jorge's slightly accented English broke into the fog of my afternoon nap. I opened my eyes to see his friendly face.

"Jorge! You came to see me! Mom, come meet my friend."

"How are you, Scott?" He sighed heavily. "I have come to say good-bye," he said softly. "Things are not working out at the home of my host family. I am returning to Costa Rica in a few days."

"In the middle of the school year?" My mother drew in closer. "Why?"

"My hosts say I do nothing. I clean dishes, help clean house, and do what I can, but it is still not enough for them. They are crazy people."

Then I had an idea, my first positive thought since the accident.

"Mom, can he stay with us? Can he come back to Skaneateles with me?"

Suddenly, the prospect of going home didn't seem quite so bleak—not with Jorge there. He was a lot of fun, so maybe things wouldn't be so bad after all.

"You would do that?" The look of hope on Jorge's face changed his whole countenance. "But you don't know me."

"It seems like the right thing to do," Mom said. "Let's go talk to your sponsors."

When my mom gets a notion to do something, especially for her kids, there's no holding her back. By suppertime, she was back at the hospital. It was obvious that she'd had an adventure beyond the blizzard she'd battled through to see me.

"Those people are really strange, Scott," she said. "When I came to the door, the husband opened it a crack and then slammed it shut. Now, here I am, in a blizzard, trying to inquire about Jorge, and they slammed the door in my face! It's a good thing you lived ten houses away. I don't know what I would have done otherwise."

Mom continued her tale. She and Jorge went to the Hatchst's to call his parents. While Mom was getting agreements and making arrangements for him to finish the school year in Skaneateles, Jorge had returned to his hosts' place and started sneaking his stuff out of the house.

"The man threatened to call the police on us, but we were determined," she said. "Once we received parental permission, we went to the courthouse and filed custody papers on Jorge's behalf."

The next day, Mom took him home to get him settled in. I was more than ready to leave the hospital when they came back to get me. Again, I wore a cast from my toes to the top of my thighs.

A few days after I got home, I was lying on my bed one afternoon, thinking about what Dr. Godfrey told me. "Scott, we've repaired your knee again, but it may never be strong enough for your sport. I strongly recommend that you give up competitive skating."

I couldn't comprehend what he told me. Not skating wasn't an option because I was fully committed to the sport. As I lay on my bed contemplating my future, Jorge knocked gently on the door.

"Yeah," I croaked. I didn't realize I'd been crying.

"Scott, may I come in?"

I quickly wiped away my tears.

"Yeah. Come on in."

"Why is it dark in here?"

"I feel down right now."

"But it is a beautiful day outside. Snow is on the ground. It is the first time I've ever seen snow."

I stared blankly at him for a moment.

"Scott, it is good to be alive today."

"Maybe for you," I grumbled. "You're following your dream."

"And you are not?"

"Dr. Godfrey says I shouldn't skate."

"Are you going to let other people dictate how you feel?"

"What?"

"If I believed my patrons, I would be back in Costa Rica now. But I did not. And now I have a new family and new friends."

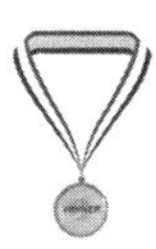

Jorge was right! For the past four days I'd been listening to people tell me what I couldn't do. But Dr. Godfrey didn't say I *couldn't*; he said I *shouldn't*. I had forgotten the most important thing: I was the one who decided whether I would ever skate again or not.

Chapter 9

Recovery

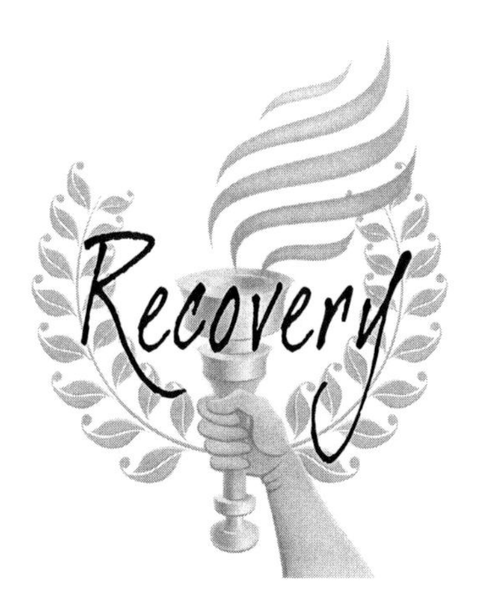

Jorge, Don, and I were pretty much inseparable during those closing months of 1976 and the first half of 1977. The bonds we forged between us helped me heal and regain my strength so I could skate again. We helped each other turn bad times into good ones, while building memories and generally enjoying high school.

At sixteen, I found myself involved in various new things at Skaneateles High School during my recovery months, including sharing a car with Bee Gee. Since he was away at college, the car was pretty much mine.

It was a 1963 F-85 Cutlass convertible, with red bucket seats in the front and a back seat roomy enough for me to install speakers from an old stereo system. I positioned them in the back so they could double as armrests. For ultimate versatility, when I parked the car with the top down, I placed the speakers on the trunk so everyone could hear the music. Despite my cast, I became the designated driver after just about every event. I accomplished this feat by grabbing my right pant leg to pull my foot up onto the dashboard so I could maneuver the pedals with my left foot.

Of course, we couldn't just have a cool interior, so Don and I also did some bodywork on the car, removing rust and restoring it to its pristine white condition. We also did some engine work and had it running smooth and rich. Once the car was in tip-top shape, we dubbed it Whitey.

School was equally interesting, especially after some drama club kids pulled us into a parody they did on "The Gong Show," a popular seventies television program. I played one of the judges, Jorge was the second one, and Don's girlfriend was the third. Don and his brother, the obvious winners, played in a fifties band. I don't know whether it was the band or the song "Teenager in Love" that earned them the winning slot, but they did a good job. The saxophone player was awesome.

Our ninety minutes of high school fame set the tone for the rest of the year, especially for Jorge, who started hanging around the drama kids all the time. With his upbeat personality, he fit right in; indeed, it was hard to stay down when Jorge was around. He liked to be around people, especially girls.

Since I wasn't spending all my time practicing or studying, I had time to date a girl named Cindy, whose dad was the superintendent of schools. Don, Jorge, and I would double- and triple-date at football games, wrestling matches, and the movies.

Unlike my encounter with Butch in middle school, my sport seemed to be much more acceptable in the eyes of my high school peers. I was equally comfortable with the athletes on the football and wrestling teams as I was with the girls in my class.

As great as those times were, they didn't take the place of skating. I managed to find time to work on strengthening my leg so I could get back to the rink. Despite his reservations, Dr. Godfrey told me that there were certain exercises I had to do in my self-rehab environment. So I did them, even when I didn't feel like it; such was the discipline of training.

As I got stronger, I knew convincing the doctor that I was ready for competitive ice skating was not going to be easy. But first, I had to get my mom on board. My final push came during our last drive to Rochester to see Dr. Godfrey.

"Mom, I'm not going to break my knee again," I said. "I'll be careful."

"Scott, I'm not sure you know how to be careful."

Of course she would think that. She always reminded me that I was like a bull in a china shop, especially when we were walking in a mall or on a sidewalk. I somehow managed to always step on her heels. She could never figure out how I could master precision skating with razor-sharp blades yet not be able to translate that to the simple task of walking. But at this moment, I was unflappable.

"Do you think I want to go through this again? I've learned my lesson. I don't know what I'd do if I couldn't continue skating."

"Didn't you have a great time at school this year?"

"Yeah, but Jorge is going home in a few months and Don's graduating. I know I once said that I didn't like skating anymore, but that was because it hurt too much. We didn't know what was going on with my knee at the time. Besides, I'm better now, and I miss it."

"Missing it isn't enough, Scott," she said. "You'll get over it."

"But I don't *want* to get over it. I know there's more out there for me. If I don't go for it, then how will I ever know how far I could have taken it? I just feel like I could do something with it. When I'm on the ice, it's like being in a different world. I can't describe the feelings well enough. Living without skating is like missing a part of myself."

I didn't know what my mom was thinking as we pulled into Dr. Godfrey's parking lot. Getting out of the car, I only knew that my knee felt great.

When we finally got into the doctor's office, he came in and shook my hand.

"How are you doing, Scott? How are you getting along?"

I mumbled the appropriate response while he examined my leg. He bent and maneuvered it to see if it was healing correctly.

"You're doing very well," he said. "Do you know how lucky you are?"

"So when can I start skating again?"

"I wouldn't recommend it," he said.

"But if I did, what could I do?"

Mom stood by the door, arms folded, like she was waiting for the other shoe to drop. Dr. Godfrey addressed his comments to her instead of me.

"Certainly he shouldn't be picking in the ice for a jump with that leg," Dr. Godfrey said.

"That's understandable," I said, ignoring the fact that he wasn't looking at me.

"Since it's happened twice with that bone," he continued slowly, "even with the screw and repair, it is susceptible to breaking. So he should stay away from that type of movement. Are you seriously considering this, Mrs. Gregory?"

"Continue, please," Mom said quietly.

"He should keep from pounding and twisting the knee," he continued.

"There goes my free-skating," I mumbled, feeling like I was being talked about, despite my presence in the room.

"And no jumps," Dr. Godfrey was on a roll now, "nothing that would put too much pressure on those joints."

By the time he finished his ever-growing list, it became clear that I would not be able to free-skate. Ice dancing seemed to be my best option. That way, I could at least continue competing in my sport, which was all I really wanted to do.

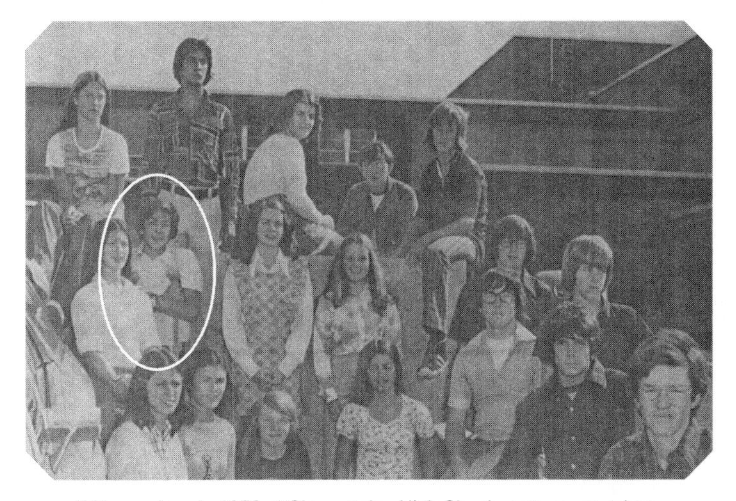

With my class in 1976 at Skaneateles High Shool - note my crutches

CHAPTER 10

New Partner

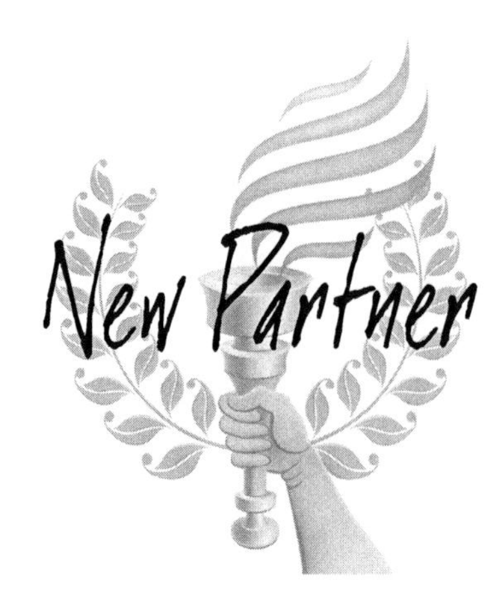

Once my mother reluctantly agreed to my decision, I was anxious to get back to Buffalo. I just knew that summer would drag on forever, but thankfully, it didn't. Jorge returned to Costa Rica, so it was just Don and me, along with our girlfriends. That last summer went by all too fast as we spent a lot of time on the lake in my dad's boat. Then Don was off to school, and it was almost time for me to return to Buffalo.

"Mom, I just talked to Richard," I said, joining her on the patio one afternoon. A warm breeze rippled the lake's waters. Mom looked up from her book.

"What did he say?"

"He's on board with the ice dancing. He's going to start interviewing partners."

"You're sure this is what you want?"

"Yeah. Being off the ice for two years has shown me how much I love it. I've got to see how far I can take it." I sat in a chair across from her. "I'll always wonder what I could have done if I walk away now."

"But Nationals are just over six months away, and you don't even have a partner yet."

"I know it's a long shot, Mom, but it's the only one I've got."

"All right," she sighed. "You've just got to be smart and careful. I don't want to see you hurt again."

Richard called me a few days later. I was going to stay with the Gebhardts, a local family with strong ties to the Buffalo Skating Club. He had also put out feelers to see who was willing to work with me. My two-year absence made me virtually unknown in the ice-dancing world. With the list of potential partners narrowed to three, Richard felt that the best fit was Judy Ferris, a national competitor in her own right.

Finally, it was time for me to leave. Cindy promised to come and see me compete, but I didn't really expect to see her anytime soon. Because I was stepping back into the zone, nothing else mattered as much as my training.

As much as I would have liked to take Whitey, my folks decided I needed transportation that would handle a heavier driving schedule than the twelve-year-old Cutlass, so I inherited one of the family cars and drove to Buffalo. When I arrived at the Gebhardt's house, I noticed that the roofline interrupted itself with multiple gables. I parked behind a white Camaro with "SKITS" on the license plate, which made me wonder where Richard had placed me. Getting past my trepidation, I headed toward the front door. Before I could knock, a petite, high-energy, no-nonsense lady stepped out on the stoop. Her name was Helene Gebhardt, better known by those who love her as "Lady."

"So, you're Scott," she said.

"Yes, ma'am. That's me."

"You're smaller than I thought," she replied.

"I'm tall enough," I said, pulling my 5' 8 ½" frame as high as I could, wishing I could grow a few more inches right before her eyes.

"Come on in, and welcome to my house," she said, stepping back from the doorway. "Follow me. I'll take you to your room. It's my son's, but he's in college now."

Practically running upstairs, she led me to a huge room with a bed, bureau, and desk. Glow-in-the-dark stars dotted the vaulted ceiling, which reminded me of my old room at home. Her house wasn't messy, but it was "lived in," so I felt very comfortable there. I couldn't have found a better home away from home. I settled in quickly, eager to get back into training.

Wanting to make a good impression on my new partner, I arrived at Nichols Rink early. Located on the campus of a private school, this rink was the home of the Buffalo Skating Club. Entering the building from the crisp, September afternoon, the first thing I noticed was the cavernous, musty, old smell common to this type of facility. Although I was confident that I would get there before Judy, I was surprised to see her practicing to the left of the snack bar.

I put on my skates and joined her on the other side of the rink. It was obvious that we were well matched in every way. At about 5' 4" with light-brown hair, she looked like she could have easily been a member of my family.

"Hey, Judy!" I said, gliding toward her.

She looked up. "Hey, yourself." She tossed that remark over her shoulder, so I couldn't tell whether it pleased her or not.

"Uh, yeah," I replied. "Have you seen Richard?"

"He's up in his office," she said. I looked up toward the glassed-in gallery, which housed the rink's VIP room and various offices. Richard's was in the back left corner, the only one with drawn curtains.

"He said he'd be back in about fifteen minutes. He suggested that we warm up." She hesitated a moment, then she got this funny look in her eye. "Should I call you Scott, or do you prefer Gimp?"

I laughed at her remark, relaxing a bit. We took some time getting to know each other, slowly gliding around the rink side by side.

"Richard says you're still in high school," she said.

Even though I was enrolled as a senior at Amherst High, I somehow knew that it wouldn't be the carefree social scene I had enjoyed at Skaneateles. "Yeah, well, I guess you're not."

"I'm a freshman at the university, studying criminology, just like my boyfriend," she said. "I think it helps to have similar interests, don't you?"

Before I could answer, Richard arrived and started to put us through the paces. The playfulness that danced through Judy's eyes moments earlier was gone. She was now all business. Her number-one rule was "No goofing off while training."

The practice was intense. I was still stiff with a leg that needed to be strengthened. As a result, I had only a limited range of motion and mobility on the ice. I don't know which was more frustrating: the embarrassment of being so clumsy and stiff or pushing to get past the awkward pain without hurting myself again.

My days quickly settled into a routine. I started dating a girl named Amy, Lady's next-door neighbor. I helped Lady when I could by mowing the lawn, raking the leaves, washing the car, and doing chores around the house; but I was focused on preparing for Regionals, which was less than two months away. Then Lady decided to help me with one of my hidden weaknesses.

"Scott, come here," she said after I came in from raking the leaves.

"Yes, ma'am," I replied, walking to her.

She handed me a piece of paper. "Learn these."

Lady had neatly printed twenty words on a 3 x 8 piece of paper.

"Learn them how?" I was confused.

"Learn to spell them," she said as she started to walk away. "Good communicators must be able to spell."

Discussion ended, case closed. Every week I awoke to find a new list of words on the kitchen table by the touch light. Spelling aside, Judy and I focused on becoming partners.

As the first ones on the ice most mornings, we went over our routines and practiced the dances. At the time, I didn't think twice about the repetition. It wasn't difficult to do a three-and-a-half minute program packed with lifts and dancing. We worked on sections over and over and ran through the whole program again and again. My leg strengthened more, so my range of motion increased.

Then it was time for our first competition, the North Atlantic Regionals. We had the home-court advantage, since it was held at Nichols. We didn't win, but we did come in second, which was a good showing considering our short time together. We hoped things would turn around at the Eastern Sectionals in Philadelphia, but everything seemed to be stacked against us when we awoke that snowy Monday morning.

"Scott, they're here!" Lady's message greeted me halfway down the steps. My textbooks with the week's assignments weighted down my luggage.

"Break—"

"Don't say that," I said. "Wish me luck instead."

Lady had heard my story but was often one to throw caution to the wind. She laughed, then feigned a big sigh. "Very well, good luck. Let us know how it goes."

"Thanks!" I shouted, bounding down the sidewalk, sliding on the quickly accumulating snow. Richard and his wife, Mandie, were in the front seat. After I stowed my gear in the trunk, I joined Judy in the back seat.

"Should we have left earlier?" Normally, I'm relatively calm before an event, but not this time. "What if we miss our practice time?"

"We'll be fine," Richard said as he pulled into the practically empty street. "We have plenty of time."

We inched our way to Philly. I tried to push the event out of my head and engage in the small talk that seemed to drone from the front seat. Judy was taking a catnap while I kept checking my watch.

What's wrong with you? Cut it out! My mind's voice started arguing with my fly-away emotions. *If you keep this up, you're bound to worry yourself crazy.*

"Do you think we'll be there on time, Richard?"

"We'll be fine, Scott. We're not the only ones stuck in the snow. You'll get your practice time in."

"But, what if . . ."

A glance at Richard's profile told me that any further questions would be a mistake, so I tried to follow Judy's lead and nap. Instead of rest, however, dreams of skating toward an imaginable goal that I never quite reached tortured my brain. Regardless of the torment, I remained asleep, unaware of the severe snowstorm that pelted Richard's car.

When we finally arrived at the Wissahickon Figure Skating Club located on the northern borders of Philadelphia, we had just enough time to suit up and practice. I felt better—stronger than before—and ready for the competition.

My knee didn't bother me at all as we practiced our compulsories and free dance. After our session, Richard took us back to the hotel that we called home for the rest of the week.

"Meet you in the restaurant in half an hour," Judy said after check-in.

This is it! Thoughts danced idly through my mind. *This is what I've been missing.* Then Mom's warning to "be smart and be careful" intruded into my excitement, and I chuckled.

"What's so funny?" Judy asked as she unlocked the door of her room, which was across the hall from mine.

"Nothing," I replied. "I was just thinking of something my mom said."

"Oh. Meet you in half an hour." Her door shut behind her. I stepped into my room, opened my suitcase, took out my textbooks, and tossed them onto the little round table by the window. I then lay on my bed and started revisiting the routines we'd be performing during the days ahead. My eyelids drifted shut until the phone's shrill ring jolted me out of my meditation.

"Scott! Where are you?"

Judy's agitation shook me.

"What? I must have—"

"I'm at the restaurant! You said we'd meet in half an hour."

"Right."

Moments later, I was sitting with Judy, Richard, and his wife in the Polynesian-styled restaurant connected to the hotel. Somehow pineapples and leis didn't seem to fit with the snow motif that nature painted on the other side of the windows.

I managed to get my suitcase off the other bed before my parents showed up on Thursday, the first day that Judy and I competed. Despite my best intentions, my textbooks were never moved from their spot on the table. Our days were spent observing the competition and practicing our routine. Then it was our turn on the ice before family, friends, and skating aficionados who gathered to watch.

Feeling strong, confident, and determined not to do anything stupid, I knew that I just needed to focus on my skating. Our main competition was the team that won Regionals. Our performance was solid, but so was theirs.

While chatting with Richard by the bleachers, I saw the referee on the far side of the rink post the winners' names in our event.

"Come on," I said to Judy as I broke into a half-run to see where we placed.

Moments later, we joined the gaggle of skaters surrounding the board.

"Go ahead, Scott," Judy said. "You're taller. You can see the board better."

I pressed in closer to the board and skimmed the names in third and second places. Then I slowly lifted my eyes to the named winners: Judy Ferris and Scott Gregory. I turned to Judy with a big grin plastered on my face. She looked puzzled. I lifted my index finger and nodded my head. She started doing "the Judy quick-step" right there. Richard stepped in behind her and quickly joined in the celebration.

Then it came time for the winners to come forward and receive their medals. Judy and I glided out to the podium. As we received our medals, I glanced into the bleachers and saw my parents standing on their feet, grinning bigger than ever. My mom looked like she was laughing and crying at the same time. As we stepped onto the center block on the podium, I noticed Richard, who couldn't have been prouder. Yet, I didn't miss the long shot. The next stop was Nationals in Portland, Oregon, only a month away.

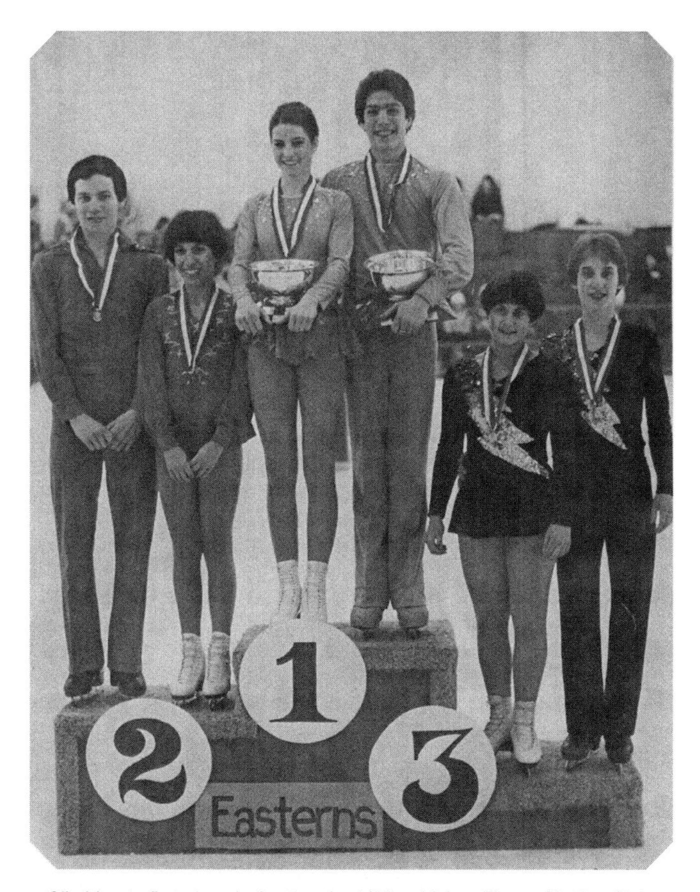

Climbing to first place in Sectionals at Wissahickon Figure Skating Club,
Judy and I qualify to compete at our first national championship.
Left: Philip Piasecki & Susan Costantino (silver); right: Terri Slater & David Lipowitz (bronze)

CHAPTER 11

Nationals

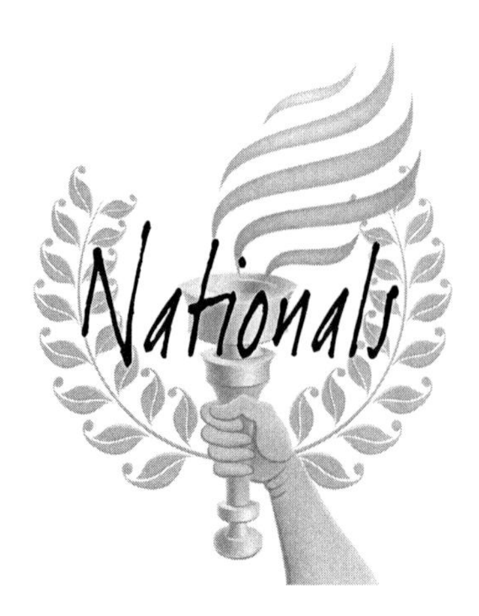

We were on our way to Nationals before we knew it. Judy was especially wide-eyed and overwhelmed. For me, it was just another cool adventure.

As Buffalo residents, we were used to cold weather, but Portland was different. It was cold—and wet. Its elevation and perpetual overcast gave us the sense that we were walking inside a cloud. As dreary as the outside seemed, inside our hotel it was like a big party. When we entered the lobby, we were directed to tables where we signed in, got our pictures taken, picked up our badges and schedules, and received gifts from sponsors.

I noticed that Judy was acting a little strange, but I simply tried to ignore it. We were, after all, at the U. S. Figure Skating Championships. In less than six months, after almost two years off the ice, I was back in the game.

But Judy would not be ignored. She revealed her master plan at breakfast the next morning.

"Scott, please pass the orange juice." I absent-mindedly handed Judy a juice carafe. As I watched her pour the deep orange liquid, I realized that she had been drinking something different moments earlier.

"Didn't you just have grapefruit juice?" I'd never known Judy to be so food-conscious.

"I'm going to eat and drink healthy if it kills me," she said just before she gulped down the large glass of juice. "You should be more careful about what you eat. This is too important." She firmly set the empty vessel on the table.

"I don't know," I muttered. "I do just fine."

"That's silly," she said. "I'm going upstairs for my gear. See you in a few minutes."

I looked at Richard, who sort of shrugged his shoulders as he polished off the last of his Belgian waffles. "Are you ready?"

"As I'll ever be," I said.

"Do you have your skates, your—"

"I have everything I need," I said, surprised by my own agitation. Richard looked puzzled.

"Is something eating you, Scott?"

"No, I'm fine. I'll get my gear." Before Richard could ask anything else, I was up and out of my chair. At seventeen, I thought he'd give me a little more credit.

My annoyance quickly passed as the prospect of skating in my first national level competition hit me. A half hour later, we were at Lloyd Center. Walking into the massive lobby with multiple avenues into the rink, the reality of the task ahead hit both Judy and me. There was no musty smell here.

"This is amazing," she exclaimed, once we were through the double doors onto the rink. "It's huge!"

Richard stepped up behind us.

"Well, kids, this is it," he said. "Go warm up."

We were due on the ice in an hour, so we found a corner where we could start doing our stretches. Suddenly, Judy stopped.

"Scott, I don't think I feel so good."

"What?" I couldn't believe it.

"Maybe this healthy eating is undoing me. I'll be right back."

She jumped up and ran to the girl's bathroom. Richard saw her leave and quickly joined me.

"What's wrong with Judy?" He looked concerned.

"Too much of a good thing," I replied vaguely. "She'll be right back."

Moments later Judy returned, looking a bit shaken and somewhat pale, but there was no doubt that she would perform. After warming up, we headed to the locker room to change our clothes and put on our skates. Returning to the rink, we saw onlookers filtering in for the afternoon's competition. That was our cue to go into the waiting area under the bleachers where we could prepare mentally for what was coming next. Richard followed.

Judy started pacing back and forth. Richard stood silently with his arms crossed while I leaned against the wall and started mentally revisiting the routine. We stood out in the hallway for what seemed like hours. Richard glanced at his watch and quietly stepped through the doors.

Moments later, he returned.

"You're up next," Richard said softly as he stepped back to make way for our entrance. Once we were rink side, we slipped off our blade guards, took a deep breath, and skated into place. I could hear Judy's breath catch as she looked toward the bleachers. For an afternoon event, the seats were scattered with people who had come to watch the junior compulsories. The vastness of the complex seemed overwhelming.

The familiar first notes of the dance music pushed out our awareness of the crowd as all the moves in my head came to life. The hours of practice paid off as we hit the mark every time. When the music stopped, we again became aware of the audience. Polite applause signaled their approval of our performance.

"We did it! One down!" I said to Judy with a big grin.

"This is incredible!" she replied as we took our bows and skated off the ice, making room for the next performers.

We watched the numbers closely, and by the end of the compulsories, we were in a solid first place. Ready for a break, Judy and I picked up our gear and headed for the bus when we heard an unfamiliar voice call my name.

Walking briskly toward us, the tall, slender man seemed excited. "What a performance!" he said as he grabbed my hand and started shaking it.

"Thank you, sir," I said. Judy stood beside me, beaming.

He took a step back and stared at us for a moment, studying us like a connoisseur would view a great painting in a museum. Then he spoke.

"And you two have only been together six months?"

"Yes, sir," I replied. Now that he was closer, I could see that he was one of the judges.

"Well, I don't know how you did it, but that's the best Rocker Foxtrot I've ever seen."

Before we could respond, he turned and walked away muttering, "Amazing, utterly amazing."

Judy and I looked at each other and giggled. This was too good. We were high on the thrill of it all.

Our final performance was set for Saturday afternoon, February 17. As we posed in the spotlight waiting for the music to begin, my mind briefly skipped to the last six months. This was what I'd been working toward. When the music started, I was immediately in the zone, totally unaware of anything but the dance until one brief moment when I lunged forward and draped Judy over my knee. Looking at her and then up, I briefly noticed the audience, fully engaged. The music, calling my gaze back to Judy to pull her up, carried us through the rest of the program.

Our reward came at the end of our high-energy performance, when the crowd's enthusiastic applause filled the rink. We knew we did well, but neither Judy nor I expected the final results that blinked onto the digital scoreboard at the event's end. We were the new junior national champions. Little did I know that this win catapulted us into a whole new level of recognition as top-level skaters.

With our victory in hand, we boarded the plane the next day and headed back to Buffalo, exhausted and exhilarated at the same time. Going home was always humbling because few outside our skating circle were aware of the impact of what we were doing. But that was all right. We knew, Richard knew, and our families knew. That's all that mattered.

"Please fasten your seat belts. We are preparing to land. Be sure to stow all luggage, place your seat in the upright position, and secure your tray."

The flight attendant's voice, combined with Judy's finger poking me in the ribs, stirred me from a very sound sleep.

"Back to reality," I mumbled as I stretched in my seat. The whine of flaps down and the wheel-skidding thump of the plane touching down notched up my awareness. "How long did I sleep?"

"You slept through dinner," Richard said, leaning forward from the seat he and his wife occupied behind us.

Judy seemed wistful as she looked at me. "Do you think your folks will be here?" Skating was an expensive sport. Not only was she going to college, but she also had to work to pay for her lessons so she could pursue her passion. Because of the expense, her parents could rarely attend any events unless they were local.

"No," I said. "We'll celebrate when I get back home."

By now the plane had stopped and we were grabbing our gear from overhead storage. Judy, Richard, his wife, and I shuffled along with the crowd when a murmuring from the people in front of us caught our attention.

"What are they saying?" Judy asked, craning to see what was ahead.

"Dunno," I replied. "Something about some celebrity on the plane." I looked around. "They were probably in first class. I guess we missed it."

"Aw, gee," she complained. "It would have been neat to see a celebrity and maybe get an autograph or something."

As we stepped off the jetway, camera lights started flashing, and a local news reporter stuck a microphone in front of our faces. Looking around, Judy and I saw both sets of parents looking on and grinning. We looked at each other and started laughing. I guess we were the celebrities! After all, we were national champions.

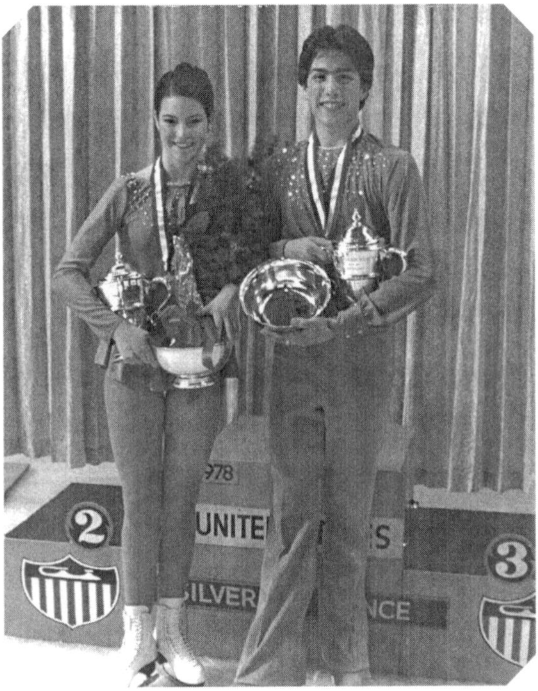

Judy and I with our trophies, winning the 1978 Junior Dance Championship in Portland, Oregon.

Chapter 12

A League of Our Own

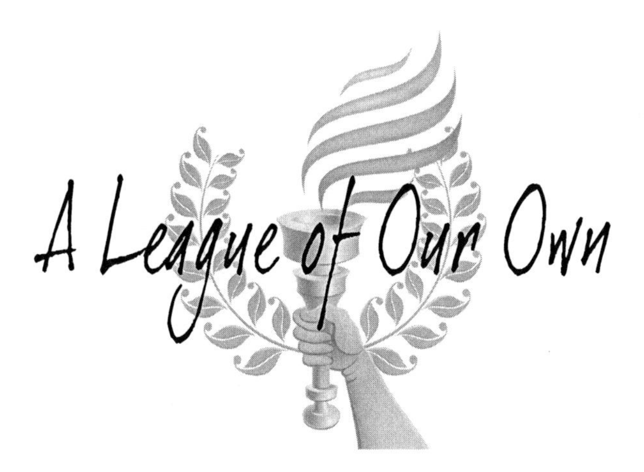

As junior national champions, we became local celebrities and were invited to perform in exhibitions and shows. One of our most exciting invitations was to participate in the elite Olympic Training Camp in Squaw Valley, California, home of the 1960 Winter Olympics.

While we found the experience at Nationals exhilarating, stepping off the airplane at Reno, Nevada, carried us into a whole new world that was much more sophisticated than upstate New York. There were slot machines in the airport. I thought it was funny that you could gamble while waiting for your luggage.

Richard, Judy, and I rode a school bus from the airport to Squaw Valley. It seemed odd to be taking such a bumpy ride along with the top national skaters who were all there for one reason—to improve in their sport.

Stepping off the bus onto the grounds of Squaw Valley made you feel like you were in an Olympic Village. Athletes and coaches walked around casually between the dormitories, cafeteria, and the practice rink.

We quickly settled into the dorm and started scouting out the camp. "This is going to be so good," Judy said as we wandered around the grounds. "I can't believe we're really here."

"Yeah," I said softly, eager to get started. "This is great."

"Oh, my gosh!" Judy said, stopping in her tracks. "Look over there!"

"Where?" I saw another couple walking on the far end of the quad.

"That's, that's . . ." I saw two rival skaters in what appeared to be an intense conversation.

"Come on, Judy. We're gawking."

"But Scott, they're . . ."

"Here for the same reason we are. It's getting late. We'd better head on back."

I slept well that night. It was the beginning of a new chapter; I just knew it.

The next morning, the crisp mountain air smelled clean and felt refreshing. After breakfast in the cafeteria, we moved tables and chairs along the walls to clear a space for our first class of the day.

"I can't believe we're really here," Judy said while we waited for our teacher to arrive.

"I can't believe we're here, either. I can't wait to get to the rink," I said. "This is different."

Our conversation halted when a tall, lanky, dark-haired lady with spiky short hair burst into the room.

"Gather round everyone," she said as she dropped her bag on the floor by the door. "I'm going to teach you something new, different, and fun. It's called the energy ball."

"The what?" Judy whispered.

I looked around the room and didn't see anything that remotely resembled a ball.

"This is an energy ball," she said as she placed her hands around a small, imaginary ball positioned at her midriff. "I want each of you to identify your energy ball and hold it in front of you."

"This is so not real," I whispered to Judy as I formed an invisible baseball in front of me. After a few snickers from various parts of the room, everyone wrapped their hands around unseen balls of various sizes and shapes.

"Now, place that little ball inside your body and discover how it rolls around in different parts of your body—from your left shoulder to your arm, up your elbow, down into your belly and into your leg"

"What?" I didn't think I heard her correctly.

"Scott, this is so cool!" Judy giggled as she pressed her hands against her stomach.

"You're sure?"

"Try it, silly," she said. And then she was gone, her eyes closed. She was obviously on a journey with her imaginary ball.

So I tried it. I wrapped my mind around the imaginary ball and watched it disappear from in front of my midriff to inside. Suddenly, I was translated into a new realm, discovering a new way of engaging my body that promised to move me to even greater possibilities in the world of ice dancing.

As I was doing it and getting the hang of it, the teacher acknowledged me.

"Oh, good, Scott. You've got it." To the class, she pointed out, "He's doing good."

I smiled and continued my energy ball journey. All too soon, our encounter was over. It was time to head to the rink, so we rushed back to our rooms, gathered our gear, met with our group, and went to the rink.

"This is more like it," I said as I sat on a bench in the lobby. Left foot first and then my right, I laced up my skates. I don't know how she did it, but Judy was already inside, gazing at something outside the rink.

"Look at the view," Judy said as I joined her inside the rink. Her voice was tinged with awe.

"What view?" I asked. Then I noticed that the rink's fourth side, which was open, offered a panorama of snow and ice-covered mountains. It was more vivid than the picture postcards we'd seen in the gift shop. For a moment, we were stunned by the beauty of creation right in front of us that was more majestic than art could ever render. "Whoa!"

That moment quickly snapped closed when a man's voice called the ten teams to gather around him. Judy and I grabbed hands and skated over to the other nine teams who were also warming up on the ice.

"Okay, everyone, gather round." The coach's gentle yet gruff voice pulled all the stragglers in. "I'm Ron Ludington, but most people call me Luddy. I competed here in the 1960 Olympics, and I teach out of Wilmington, Delaware. My job today is to teach you a new dance, which I call 'The Yankee Polka.'" For the next hour, we learned the basics of Luddy's original fifty-two step, quick-moving dance that was part of the following year's compulsories.

The rest of the week rushed by as we worked with different coaches, learned new material, and were generally equipped with techniques we needed to know to effectively compete at the seniors' level. The three of us returned home, excited. We had been introduced to new concepts, fresh ideas, and a different way of doing things. A few weeks later, I graduated from high school. Then, I enrolled at Buffalo State College and casually continued my studies.

Judy and I were optimistic about Nationals. The first step, of course, was Regionals, so our daily activities centered around practice.

It was a typically cold and hazy morning in upstate New York. Judy and I again were the first ones at the rink, so we had the ice to ourselves. Richard was upstairs, in his office. After spending some time warming up, it was time to work on our compulsory dances.

"Ready for the Yankee Polka?" I asked as we got in position. Judy nodded her head. We started the music. Skating backwards with Judy snuggled in close, we were hip to hip. Everything seemed right, just like Luddy taught us, until we both kicked backwards. Judy's heel dug right into my shin.

"Oh, my gosh!" I stopped. I knew something had happened, but I didn't know what.

"What did I do?" Judy asked as she pivoted around. "Did I hit you? How badly?"

All color drained from Judy's face. She was almost as pale as I felt.

I knelt to assess the damage. My pant leg didn't rip, but I knew something was wrong. I rolled it up and discovered a one-inch hole in my shin that just missed the bone. I put my arm around Judy's shoulder, and she helped me hobble off the ice.

When I took my boot off, blood gushed out. Judy grabbed a towel, wrapped it around my leg, and then ran up to get Richard. Moments later I was in his car and on my way to the hospital.

The doctors said that Judy's blade cut through the membrane that holds the muscle in place. Since it was particularly sensitive to stitching, this meant I had to stay off the ice for three weeks to let it heal, which took us out of the competition for Regionals.

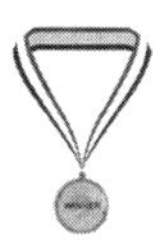

As the previous year's junior national champions, Judy and I were allowed a bye into Eastern Sectionals at Rochester. After weeks off the ice and less than a month to prepare, it was time to get in the groove. We used our time well, and a few days before our departure, we knew that we looked good. But were we good enough?

We came in a strong third at Eastern Sectionals, which wasn't bad for our first seniors' competition, as well as coming off an injury. Since our coach convinced us that we would do well at Nationals in Cincinnati, Ohio, we were looking forward to also going to the World competition in Vienna, Austria.

But Vienna just didn't happen for us. We came in tenth, despite Richard's assurances. We may have been at the top of our game as juniors, but we learned that we had a long way to go before we'd be competitive seniors.

After our disappointing placement at Nationals, I entered my year of discontent. It seemed like Richard and I were butting heads all the time. Nothing I did ever seemed to satisfy him.

We never seemed to be able to regain our position. Despite our dismal record, we were invited to Squaw Valley again. The more I worked with other coaches, the more I knew I needed to make a change. But the change was hard. Richard was the one who took me beyond the borders of Skaneateles. He stayed with me through my injuries and always seemed to be there for me.

Yet I was frustrated because he still treated me like I was the twelve-year-old he took into his home. But I wasn't; I was nineteen and wanted to be independent. Amy, my sounding board and greatest supporter, was most likely the only one who knew how I really felt. She helped me keep myself together, regardless of my frustration level.

Everything came to a head in 1979 at the National Sports Festival in Colorado Springs. Because I knew Richard so well, I understood how to push his hot buttons, which I did often—even when I really didn't want to. It became so evident that he walked away from us in the middle of the competition.

Judy knew that things had grown tense between Richard and me.

"Scott, are you all right?" She was obviously concerned and even hurt by my demeanor.

"I'm done, Judy. This is my last competition with Richard."

Tears pooled in her eyes. "But, Scott . . ."

"No matter how hard I try to concentrate on skating, the excitement and magic is gone." I could sense the same in Judy. The magic was indeed gone.

We came in third. Since there were only three teams competing, our last-place position confirmed that I'd made the right decision.

"Scott! Where will you go?"

"I'm not sure. Probably Wilmington with Luddy. Come with me."

"I can't," Judy whispered, her voice warbling as she tried to maintain control.

"You mean you won't." I tried hard to keep an accusing tone out of my mouth.

"I can't. My family's there, my boyfriend, my school. I don't have the money to relocate."

"And Richard?"

"He's my coach, my trainer. I can't leave him."

"Your choice," I said as I walked away.

The flight home was tense. The day after we returned, I went to the rink to clean out my locker. Richard was nowhere to be seen. I said my good-byes to everyone and then returned to my home in Buffalo. Lady came into my room as I was packing.

"So you're really leaving," she said, her voice a bit gruffer than normal.

"Yeah," I replied. "And thanks to you, I can spell."

The room was quiet for a moment.

"Scott, you may be leaving this house, but you're not leaving me."

I looked at her. "What do you mean?"

"You'll not be rid of me that easily. I intend to keep an eye on you."

"I'd like that." I knew I would miss her—a lot. She was like a second mother to me.

"Well, that's settled," she said. "Come on down for some lunch before you leave. You can't drive home on an empty stomach." Then she was gone.

Through the months and years ahead, she became one of my biggest fans.

My final good-bye was to Amy, who had become my best friend during my last years in Buffalo. She later accepted a teaching position in Gaithersburg, Maryland, which was only two hours from Wilmington, Delaware, where I moved after I found a new coach. We continued to see each other for two more years until the additional time away for training and competitions caused the bond to fade.

Chapter 13

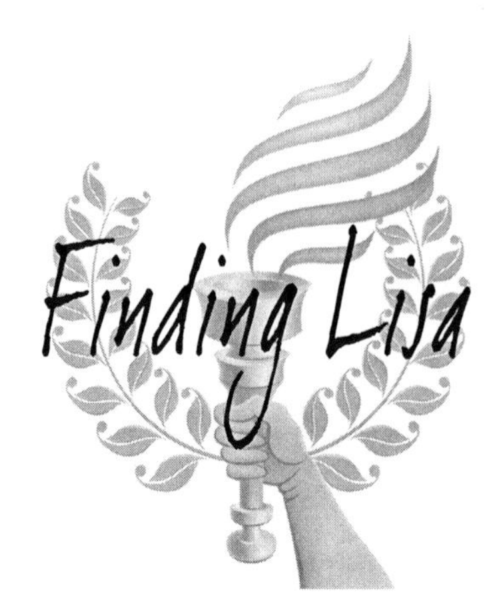

Finding Lisa

"Okay, yeah, that sounds good. I'll give her a call." I hung up the phone and added a name to the list of candidates I was interviewing.

"Scott, I'm going shopping," Mom said as she walked into the family room. "Do you need anything?"

"How about a new partner?"

"No luck yet?"

"Nope," I said, standing up and stretching.

"What about that girl you tried out with last week?"

"Renee? She's a great ice dancer, but we just didn't feel right together."

Mom looked skeptical.

"I know it was easier when Richard did everything, but I've got to do this on my own. Besides, a friend of mine just called to tell me that Lisa Spitz is looking for a new partner."

"Didn't she win junior dance at Nationals? She has a partner."

"They split. She's looking." I grabbed the phone and started dialing. Mom quietly left to run her errands.

"Hello, Lisa? I'm Scott Gregory. I heard that you're looking for a partner."

Silence greeted my introduction.

"Lisa, are you there?"

Before I could disconnect, she moved into high-speed chatter. At sixteen, she was eager to build on her success. Her enthusiasm was catching, so I arranged a meeting for the following week.

It was early in August when I drove up to Lake Placid to meet Lisa a few weeks after my twentieth birthday. I felt free for the first time in a long time, more confident and in control, especially driving in my brown Mustang II with a T bar roof and tan interior. It was my dad's idea to give me a car with a manual transmission for my high school graduation gift. Of course, he had to teach me to drive it first.

When I got to the rink, I found Lisa pacing back and forth, talking to her fellow skaters. High energy was just bouncing off her.

"Lisa?" She was bubbly, vivacious, and obviously anxious to get going. "Good, you're here," she said, practically dragging me inside. After a quick connection with Tom Lescinski, a renowned international ice-dancing coach who agreed to evaluate us, we sat on a nearby bench and laced our skates up.

After skating around the rink together for about five minutes, we got to know each other a bit. Lisa was funny. I knew right away that she was the one because it just felt right. A few basic stroking exercises later, we skated over to Tom.

"Well, what do you think?" I asked.

"Let me take a look at some dances," he said.

I felt a real chemistry between us. We agreed to do an Argentine Tango, and considering that it was our first time together, it went rather well. We just needed to get Tom's perspective.

"It works," he said. "You're well matched. Your hair coloring is close. Your hips and legs are compatible. I see no reason why this won't work."

"Thanks," I said. "We appreciate your time."

Then Lisa and I decided to have a go at The Blues, a compulsory dance we both knew. After we finished the pattern, a loud belch escaped from her mouth. She laughed out loud.

"Sorry," she said, laughing. "I belch when I'm nervous."

I was taken by surprise, but I laughed with her.

"Okay," I hesitated. "So, do you want to partner with me?"

"Are you kidding? I've always wanted to skate with you. You're a great skater. I can't believe you're picking me. I mean, I heard that—"

"Take a breath," I said, laughing. "I was thinking about going to Wilmington with Ludington."

"You're kidding! He's the best!"

"But what about your parents?"

"They're all for this. I'm ready to move, to do whatever it takes."

"Okay, I'll call you when I have something definite."

The four-hour drive home seemed to take forever. I was anxious to call Luddy and see if he would be willing to add us to his team. He just had to.

The house was empty when I arrived home. I carried my overnight bag in and dropped it on the kitchen floor. Making a beeline for the phone, I called the Skating Club of Wilmington and asked for Ron Ludington.

"Hello?"

"Yes, um, Mr. Ludington, I'm Scott Gregory. You may not know . . ."

"I know who you are. What can I do for you?"

"Um, I'm no longer with Richard Callahan, so . . ."

"I heard that you two split. What have you been doing since then?"

"Finding a new partner. Lisa Spitz and I have decided to . . ."

"Really? That could be interesting."

"Yeah, well, um, we were wondering if perhaps, maybe . . ." This was a lot harder than I thought it would be.

"You want to come to Wilmington? You want to know if I would take you on as a team?"

"Yes, sir. We are very interested . . ."

"You and Lisa are good skaters. You certainly have the talent, but do you both have the heart to take it all the way?"

He threw me off. *Did I have the heart?* There were moments when I thought about quitting due to my injuries, but my parents urged me on. I couldn't have done any of this without them.

"What do you mean?"

"It's the heart, the determination, and the drive that will take you to the top," he continued. "Be here next week."

He hung up. It was a done deal.

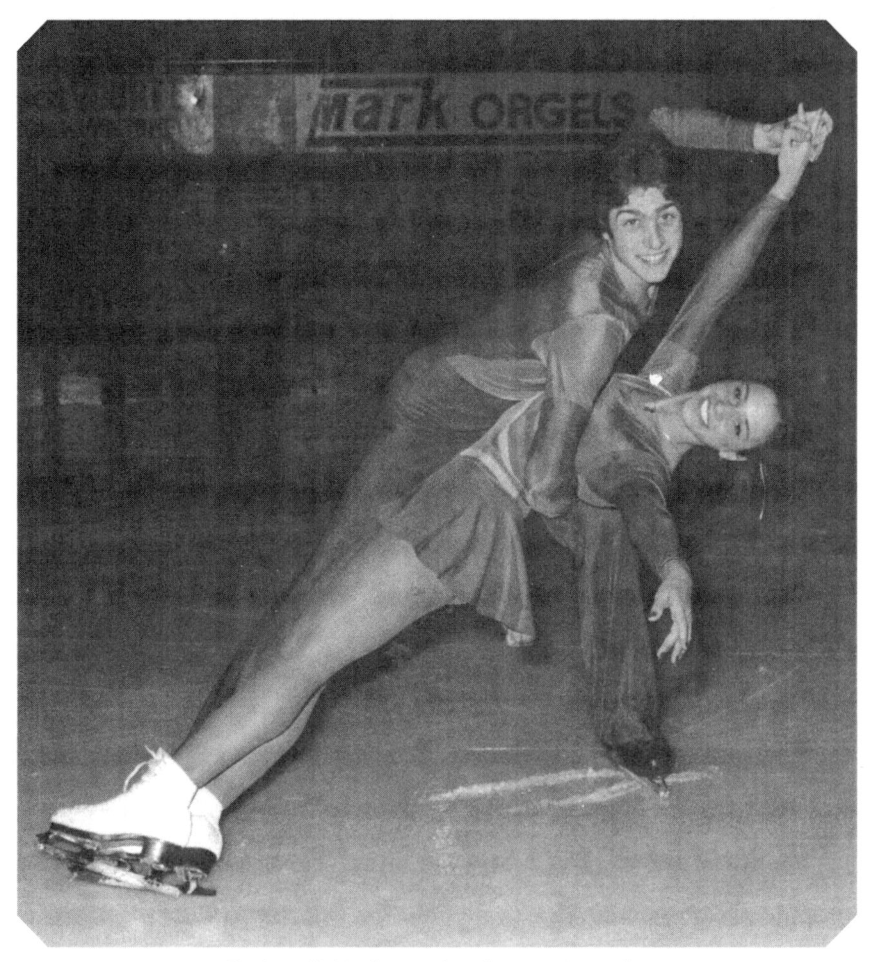

Skating with Lisa in one of our first practice outfits.

Chapter 14

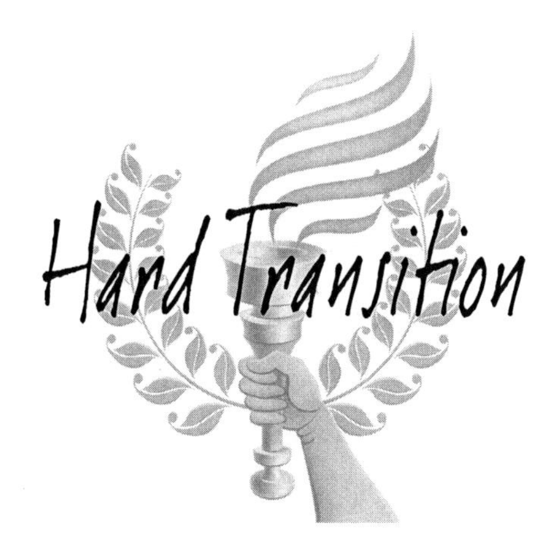

Hard Transition

I dialed Lisa's number. She picked up on the first ring.

"Lisa?"

She started screaming.

"Lisa?" Concern tinged my voice.

"We're in, we're in! I just knew it. When do we leave?"

"Wait, how did you—"

"Are you kidding?" she screamed. "I could tell by your voice."

We made plans to meet in Wilmington the following Wednesday. It was a good four and a half hour drive for me. After I finished talking to Lisa, I called the Skating Club of Wilmington and found a host family where we could stay until we could find more permanent lodging.

I arrived at our host family's home and quickly settled into a bizarre and incredibly demanding schedule that separates the wannabes from the pros. It didn't take long to discover what Luddy was talking about. Lisa and I were like little fish in a big pond, training with top skaters like the current national dance champions and the top national pair champions. This gave me a new and greater appreciation for the "survival of the fittest" concept.

When I was younger, it seemed that skating was all I needed to do to get in shape, but Luddy's regimen included off-ice training. Though not thoroughly convinced this was necessary, I half-heartedly participated in weight training, ballroom dancing, and ballet. We devoted six to eight hours a week to this training, alongside our ice time.

I never knew what my parents' arrangements were for my lessons with Luddy, but if he noticed that you weren't working hard enough or wasting time, your penalty was no lesson that day. With so many serious skaters on board, he had to invest his time wisely. This was no time to waver or wonder if you really wanted to do this because you would never survive at the championship level with that kind of wishy-washy mindset. At this level, there was only one road to travel—the road to success. At least, that was my attitude.

The Skating Club of Wilmington is an incredible facility that has been easily adapted to training world class ice skaters. But first and foremost, it is a social skating club built and maintained by the dues and contributions of its members. The national champions who train there add to the prestige, but they are expected to work around the members' schedules. That meant we didn't get on the ice until almost midnight. We would skate for ninety minutes, take a break, and then come back and skate until 5 a.m.

During our break, we could go to the lounge that overlooked the rink and work on our routines. The lounge was incredible because it had dancers' mirrors along the wall at either end. If we didn't go upstairs, we drove to Dunkin' Donuts for coffee and maybe a donut.

We finished practice and went home to sleep while most people were having their breakfast. By noon, we returned to the rink for our ninety-minute afternoon practice. Then we went to ballet or our weight lifting classes. We finished up around 5:30 p.m., went home, ate, napped, and reported back to the rink before midnight.

Within a couple of weeks, I started looking for an apartment. Very conscious of the amount of money my parents were contributing to my career, I tried to find something relatively inexpensive but close to the skating club. It wasn't in the best of neighborhoods, but at $175 a month for a studio apartment, the price was right.

I managed to live a week or so with virtually no furniture. Fully aware of my plight, my mom told me to gather some guys together because she and my dad were coming down with furniture to fill my pad.

"We should be there around noon," she said. Just hearing her voice on the telephone was reassuring. "We have the Spaulding's truck."

"I'll meet you just as you get off the Marsh Road exit from I-95."

I found three guys who were available to help unload the truck. We arrived five minutes early.

"I can't wait to see what they're bringing," I said, while we waited for them to arrive.

"Is that them?"

I glanced up to see a truck turning the bend. Furniture was stacked so high on the bed that it looked like it would fall over in a cross-breeze.

"I don't think so," I laughed. "They look more like the Clampetts on 'The Beverly Hillbillies' than—"

Suddenly, I stopped, not believing my eyes. My dad was at the wheel.

"Hang on," I said as I turned on the ignition and sprang the engine into gear. Easing my way to the front of the hillbilly procession, I slowed down to little more than a crawl. "I'd better go slow. One sharp turn and the whole thing could topple over."

I tried to keep my surging Mustang at a safe fifteen to twenty miles per hour, but neither my car nor my dad agreed. My Mustang kept trying to stall out, while my dad laid onto the horn. I increased my speed to about forty, and everybody seemed to be happier.

When Dad pulled up to my building, we gathered round and carried everything into my ground-floor apartment. Mom supervised the furniture arrangements, but it was obvious that my early eighties décor looked more like a jigsaw puzzle with major pieces missing. As usual, Mom had the perfect solution.

"Come along," she said, grabbing her purse. I followed several steps behind her, unsure of what to expect next. "It seems to me that we passed a consignment shop on the way here."

"A what?"

"A used furniture store where we can get everything we need for next to nothing."

With the experienced eye of an antique shopper and a sharp nose for bargains, my mother negotiated my purchase of a nice sixties-vintage end table (which happened to be stained green) and a mirror. We added a lamp here and an accent piece there, and my drab apartment was transformed into my home—a reflection of who I was at the time. I felt confident, independent, and entrenched enough to enjoy my new journey.

Living in my own apartment gave me a sense of freedom and responsibility. Of course, once a week I enjoyed a home-cooked meal with Lisa and her hosts, which helped me remain grounded in a family atmosphere. Otherwise, I decided when to sleep and when to work. If my friends wanted to come over after practice, they could. It was a great place to be.

For us, the season started with our routines. Richard used to be the one who picked out my dance music and choreographed our programs. I had taken all that for granted. But Luddy had far too many skaters to take on that responsibility, so our search started at the local record store.

"Scott, this one looks good." Lisa was holding an orange album with a picture of Mozart on the front.

"I'm not sure about classical. Nah! I don't think so," I said, returning to the polka records I was flipping through.

"How about this one?" she asked, holding up another with a skull on the lower left-hand side and an unborn child on the lower right. I looked closer, recognized the cover, and returned to my flipping.

"We're not going to skate to The Moody Blues. But I do like the idea."

"We've been here for two and a half hours. I can think of better things to do with my Saturdays than stand around a dusty old record store." For a moment I thought she would start stamping her foot and shaking her curls.

Eyeing a cover that looked promising, I pulled the album out, checked the back, and added it to the pile.

"All right," I said as I picked up the stack. "We can go."

I carried our purchases to the cashier, wrote a check for $437.50, then steered Lisa toward the car. I didn't like spending that kind of money and not knowing if I had anything usable, but that's what it took.

After dropping Lisa off at her host's house, I drove to my apartment, where I started the arduous task of listening to all the records. Experience told me that, when I found the right sounds, to submit them to Luddy for approval.

Finding the right music was a crucial first step in developing a winning routine. Hour after hour of dropping the needle into the record's groove to hear the first seconds of a promising piece often revealed either its potential or inadequacy. Before long, I had enough material to put together a four minute free dance and a two and a half minute original dance. Once Luddy approved our music, then I spent hours taping the record onto the reel-to-reel. This involved manually splicing or cutting the magnetic tape to join the different selections into one routine. This job took hours of tedious work but was well worth the effort. I eventually got very good at it— good enough for other skaters to pay me to mix and cut their music too.

It all started with that first season's work. I had just finished selecting the last of four arrangements I planned to splice together, when Lisa's phone call told me that it was time to pick her up so we could go see Luddy. Gathering up the albums and my car keys, I drove to her house, where she was waiting on the step out front.

"Ready?" she asked as she stepped into the passenger's seat.

"Yep," I replied.

"Do you think he'll like it?" Lisa sounded nervous. Time was running out, and we needed our music to choreograph our program.

"Why wouldn't he?" I replied.

Lisa sat there, saying nothing. Fortunately, the ride to Luddy's house was short. Pulling into the driveway of his wooded lot gave us a feeling of being in the country rather than near the heart of the city. This was our first visit to his home, just the two of us.

Lisa rang the doorbell. A few moments later, Luddy answered and invited us in to his living room. Shades of brown created a warm, cozy, and decidedly masculine atmosphere. Beside the fireplace, which occupied the left wall, my eyes caught sight of a basket of antique skates next to a stack of skating magazines. I wanted to go over to examine them, but my curiosity would have to wait.

"Follow me," he said cordially as he escorted us to his office, which was down the hall and on the left. While moments alone with Luddy were precious, like nuggets of gold, entering his office revealed even more about the man and his accomplishments. A poster from the 1960 Olympics was the centerpiece of his collection. Additional posters and photos of his champion skaters were tastefully framed and arranged on his wall. I wondered if I would ever be there. Yet we were there for business, not to daydream.

Lisa sat with her legs tucked under her in the chair, while I sat on the floor. Luddy leaned back in his office chair as I picked out the album with our first selection, put the needle on, and waited for the perfect notes to permeate the room. Hardly breathing, I watched Luddy, trying to gauge his reaction as he listened to the upbeat selection. When that piece was finished, Luddy didn't say a word. So, I put the second album on and played that selection. I repeated the process until we finished listening to all the music. As the final notes faded, he spoke.

"The first two will work," he said, "but I'm not so sure about the third one. Keep on looking." He handed over the four albums and returned to the stack of papers on his desk. We were dismissed.

"What does that mean?" Lisa asked once we were outside his house.

"It's back to the record store."

"Again?"

"You don't have to go," I said as I drove her back to her house. "I'll take care of this. We've got to practice."

My apartment was my haven until one morning when I came home after one of our late-night practices. I placed my key into the lock and opened the door. Stepping across the threshold, I felt that something was wrong before I saw it.

I dropped my bag at the door and entered the room slowly, cautiously, ready to react to the unexpected. About mid-way into the room, I looked to my right and saw a gaping hole on the coffee table positioned by my television stand. Instead of my Sony reel-to-reel recorder situated in the middle of the table, I saw a faint, dusty outline mocking me, showing me where my prized possession had been. The intruder also had grabbed the television, my stereo system, and a pile of my records.

"Great," I muttered sarcastically.

I checked the bedroom and kitchen. Everything else seemed okay.

Dialing the phone, I looked around and felt generally creepy. My apartment was no longer a haven because I didn't feel safe. Suddenly, the phone stopped ringing. My dad answered.

"I've been robbed," I said, surprised at how choked up I sounded.

"What?" he asked. "Are you all right? Were you hurt? What happened?"

"Someone broke into my apartment while I was at practice." I was fighting to retain control while my insides threatened to jump out of my skin. "They got my reel to reel, television, and stereo system."

"Have you called the police?"

"N-n-no, not yet."

"Call the police, and then get back to me."

I made the call, and two police officers arrived almost an hour later. After a brief examination, they showed me how the burglar gained access—through my ground-floor window that didn't latch tightly. They also told me that I needed to keep my curtains closed so people couldn't see what I had in my living room. They were there for an hour, dusting for prints and looking for clues.

After the officers left, I called my dad. He said he was sending me some money to replace what was stolen. He also told me to check with the landlord about security measures to prevent this from happening again.

After about a week, everything was back to normal. All went well for a month. I'd done everything the officers said. One morning, after Lisa and I had managed to get in some extra practice, I came home tired. Much to my surprise, my apartment door was ajar. I was pretty sure I didn't leave it that way.

Carefully, I opened the door, listened for signs of an intruder, heard none, and then stepped over the threshold. Like before, I sensed the disturbance before I saw it. I looked down and saw my big coin jar missing. This time they left my reel-to-reel but took my stereo system.

"Not again!"

I reached for the phone, called the police, and then called home.

"This is the second time in two months. Do the police have any leads?"

"No."

"We're going to have to make some other living arrangements for you," my dad said.

"Where?"

"Let me check into it," he said.

A few weeks later, he flew down to see me. I picked him up at the airport in Philadelphia. On the way back to Wilmington, he said he wanted me to meet someone.

"We have to deal with your living situation," he said as we drove to the outskirts of Wilmington.

"What do you mean?"

"What would have happened had you come in while the burglars were still there?" he asked. I had wondered that myself.

Before he could reply, I found the address he gave me. It was Rowley Realtors.

"We're going house-hunting," Dad said.

"What?"

After a quick introduction to Neil Rowley, the real estate agent was chauffeuring us around some of the safer areas of the city. We spent a couple of hours looking for houses until we came upon 1430 Foulk Road. It was a split-level home with red shingle siding, white shutters and a stone-faced garage, that looked as tired and saggy as I felt, but it had potential. The best room in the house was the living room that had a fireplace. Dad made an offer on the property that day.

"You're going to buy it?" I asked. "Isn't this more expensive than an apartment?"

"I'll cover the down payment, but it's up to you to make this house pay for itself," he said.

"What do you mean?" My brain seemed to be operating in a fog. "How can I make it pay for itself?"

"Roommates," he continued. "And with a number of guys living here, it's highly unlikely that your burglars will ever return."

Dad was right on all accounts. I did get roommates, among whom Peter Carruthers was one of the earliest. He quickly became one of my best friends. Peter and his sister, Kitty, had already gone to the 1980

Olympics. He was taller than I and muscular with straight brown hair. His adopted sister, Kitty, was petite, dark-haired, and temperamentally opposite of Peter, who some mistook as being a bit cocky. He wasn't. He was just confident, which was a well-earned attitude for all he and Kitty accomplished. Besides, he was funny and great to be around. Quite conveniently, Kitty was Lisa's best friend, so it all fit all together.

Right after closing on the house, my parents stayed for a week to help me fix the place up. It started out as a dirty mess, but by the time we finished with it, the house looked like a different place. I was twenty-one years old and settled in my first home. I couldn't believe it. Even though the house wasn't mine, I was living in it, and I was the boss. Life was good. I was doing what I had always wanted to do: follow my dream.

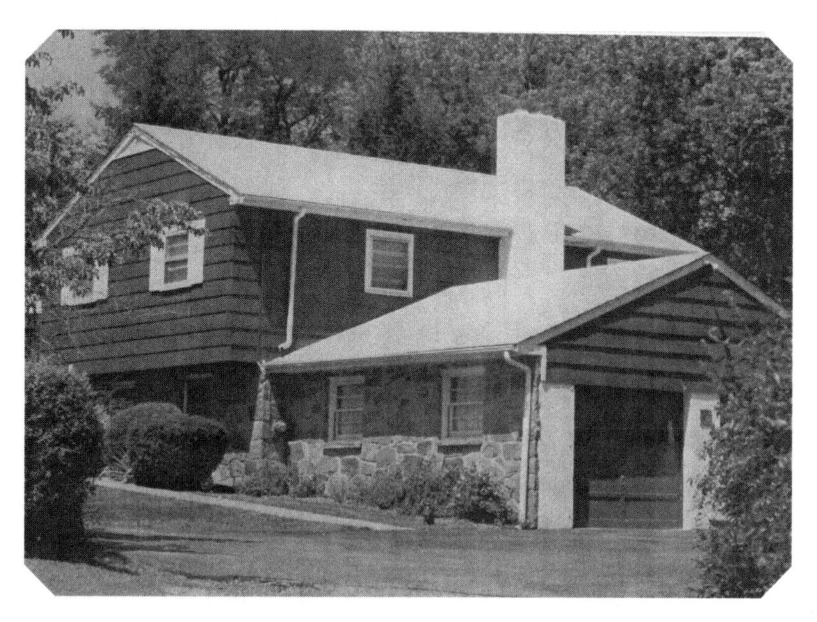

1430 Foulk Road, Wilmington, Delaware, the house I lived in and rented out to other skaters for six years. Great memories!

Chapter 15

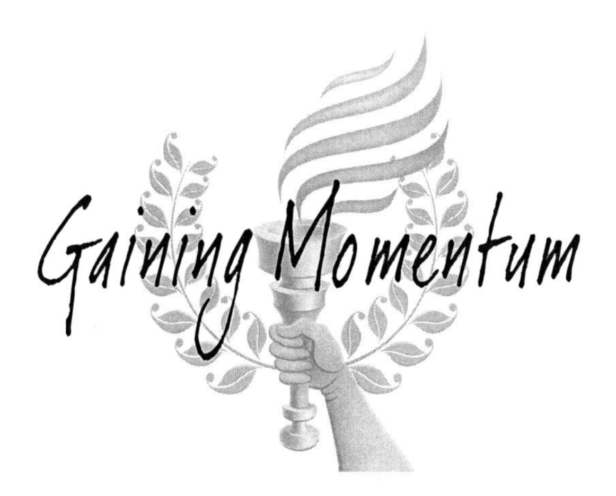

Gaining Momentum

"Mom, she's driving me nuts!" I said. It was 6 a.m. I knew that Mom was getting ready for work, but I had to talk to someone. Lisa and I had been skating together for less than two months.

"What's the problem?" I could hear my mom fixing coffee in the background.

"I'm getting tired of obstacles," I said. "Will it ever be easy?"

"Nobody said this would be easy. What happened?"

"It's not just one thing. It's . . . it's . . . well, it's like . . ." I couldn't articulate the problem. "We're just not gelling. It's like we're not focused on the same thing or moving in the same direction. I don't think she wants it bad enough."

"Honey, she's only sixteen. You're twenty. You have to give her time. You're both sacrificing a lot to move forward."

I thought about what my mother was saying. She was right about the sacrifice; the crazy hours were almost impossible to adapt to. Yet, all of Luddy's champions had to adapt. Lisa dropped out of high school and left Boston to make this work. "Okay," I mumbled, too tired to try to figure it out. "I guess you're right."

"Stick with her, Scott," Mom said. "Work it out. You're a good match. You look good together. You skate well together. Success has a way of helping things work out."

"I know," I said, not feeling as hopeful as I tried to sound. "I'd better get some sleep. I have to be back at the rink in four hours."

I tried thinking back to what I'd been like four years earlier. At sixteen, I was forced to be off the ice because of my knee. Was I being too hard on Lisa? But I quickly dismissed that thought. I knew that pushing through would take us beyond the talent and what I was hoping would take us to the top. I missed competing at the Worlds once, and I wasn't going to let it happen again. I'd just have to have enough push for the two of us.

That night we started working on our dances. At 11:30 we took the ice. We skated for an hour and a half and then took a break. We were working on our second leg at almost 3 a.m. when Lisa started complaining.

"Scott, I'm tired," she whined after we finished sections of our free-dance.

"Tired doesn't count," I said. "We have until four. Let's work longer."

"No!" she said, starting to skate to the edge of the rink. "I'm done. I'm going home."

"Lisa!" My voice sounded sharper than I intended. "You can't keep quitting! It won't work!"

"But, Sco-ottt!"

I felt like I was talking to a four-year-old.

"You said that you wanted to be the best you could be," I said. "I didn't move to Delaware just to quit before we really got started. Did you?"

Lisa skated back to me, and we worked until our training session was over. When we finished, she skated off in a huff. You're supposed to feel good about yourself after a good workout, but fighting with her drained me. I started to wonder if we would ever be on the same page.

I chose to minimize our differences, with the help of my mother and Luddy. Keeping my perspective was just as important as her pushing past fatigue and building up stamina. We were doing well at lower levels of competition, but the first opportunity to truly test our mettle came in the 1980 Nationals in Atlanta, Georgia.I thought I was pretty well-traveled at that stage of my career, but I had never seen anything like the practice rink in Atlanta. When we reached the hotel, signs directed us to a conference room to register. I looked around for a bus schedule for the practice rink but saw none.

"How are we getting to the practice rink?" I asked the registrar.

"What?" He looked confused.

"I don't see a transportation schedule for the practice rink," I said.

"Uh, you walk," he replied.

"Walk? How far is it?"

"You go to the hotel lobby and through the double doors that take you to the mall. From there you go to the courtyard, past some shops and restaurants to the rink, which is located in the middle of the Concordia."

"Really?" I was impressed. This was certainly a new concept, one that I was sure I would like.

After I finished registering, I looked for Lisa, who was on the other side of the room talking to some friends. I quickly joined them.

"Want to go see where we'll be practicing?" I asked, feeling a bit smug.

"What? How?" Lisa looked as confused as I felt a few moments earlier.

"Follow me," I said. A few others joined our small parade. Five minutes later, we were at the rink. The interior was stupefying. Thirty-story buildings surrounding the rink rose like huge columns above the ice. Laser lights undulating with different colors added to the fantasy-land ambiance.

"This is the practice rink?" Lisa said incredulously. "In a shopping mall?"

I grinned. "Yep."

While this wasn't the only practice area we used in Atlanta, it was certainly one of our favorites. Our sessions went well, an indication of what lay ahead. The competition was staged in the Omni Coliseum, a few blocks from the hotel. Throughout the week, the coliseum crowds were sparse, but the last night was another story. We were scheduled for the last event of the whole competition, yet we did not anticipate the scope of the final evening's performance. We arrived at the coliseum ninety minutes early, walked through the entrance way, and stepped into the building.

"I'll meet you out here in three minutes," I said as Lisa turned toward the women's locker room.

"Will do," she replied, trying to tone down her excitement. This was, after all, our last performance at our first Nationals. "Do you think there are many people here?"

"Dunno. Let's take our stuff to the locker rooms and then come back and look."

Moments later we met and walked toward the entrance. The closer we got, the more we started to feel it. The air was charged, and the anticipation was so real that we could almost see it surrounding us.

We stepped out to rink side and stopped. The stands were full.

"Scott?" Lisa whispered, her voice tinged with fear.

The sight of more than sixteen thousand people in the stands stunned us. The television lights and body heat from the crowd raised the arena's temperature while the ice remained cold enough to handle the evening's events. Anticipation defined the room's dynamics. For a nanosecond I couldn't move. I stood there, taking it in, realizing for the first time just how big all this was. It was a "Dorothy, we're not in Kansas anymore" moment.

"Wow," Lisa said softly. She felt it too.

"Yeah," I said. No other words found their way to my mind or my mouth.

The audience roared as the next competitors in our event made their way onto the ice. Their collective voices were indistinct but as loud as any tidal wave. That roar shook me from my paralysis. It would soon be our turn to be out there.

"Come on," I said. "We've got to get ready." I returned to the hallway where I started mentally reviewing our routine. Lisa followed and started psyching herself for our four minutes on the ice.

Too soon, but not soon enough, it was time for us to begin our final preparations before our performance.

"Come on, Lisa," I said, trying to make my voice sound naturally casual in this unnatural environment. "Let's warm up."

Like an automaton, she nodded her head and started the pre-skating stretches that promised to limber her muscles before their workout.

"Lisa?"

She kept stretching, oblivious of her surroundings.

"Lisa, it's time."

"Time for what?"

"To get ready."

"Are we really here, or am I just dreaming? There are so many people!"

"Yeah," I chuckled. "We're really here, and we're ready. We can do this."

Lisa nodded her head and took off toward her locker room. I went to mine. Moments later we returned, suited and ready to go.

"Scott! Lisa!" Luddy was motioning us into place. We joined him, took off our skate guards, and then took our place with five other teams who were waiting for their six-minute warm-ups on the ice.

"Next group of skaters, take the ice," the announcer said as we all raced on. Using the whole surface, we stroked and practiced sections of our routines, getting a feel for the surface. During our warm-ups, the audience watched and cheered. We rejoined Luddy and waited for the final call. It was not a long wait.

"Up next are Elisa Spitz and Scott Gregory," the announcer's voice echoed throughout the stadium. Like those before us, the audience roared as we skated into position while he finished the introduction. We felt good, like they really appreciated us.

As soon as the music started, we were in the zone. The audience disappeared. It was Lisa, me, the music, and the ice. It worked, and we clicked. If we thought the audience's response was loud before we started, it was cataclysmic when we finished. That confirmed what we felt. We had done well; we just didn't know how well.

Out of twenty teams in our category, Lisa and I came in sixth, which made us the second alternates to the Olympic team. This was better than Judy and I did after being together for two years. I knew I had made the right decision to change coaches before, but moving from tenth with Judy to sixth with Lisa proved it. I was climbing the mountain and enjoying the view. And there was still more to come.

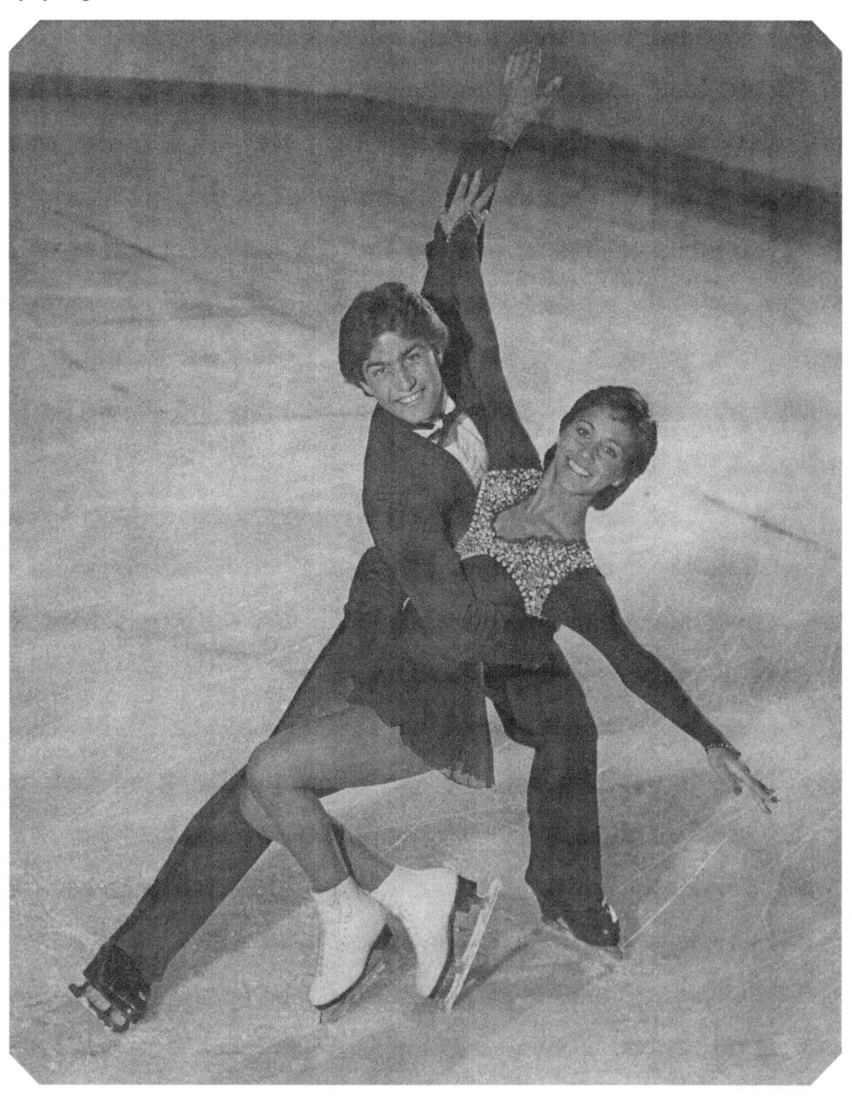

Posing with Lisa in our compulsary dance outfits,
later worn at the 1980 Nationals in Atlanta, Georgia.

Chapter 16

Competing Internationally

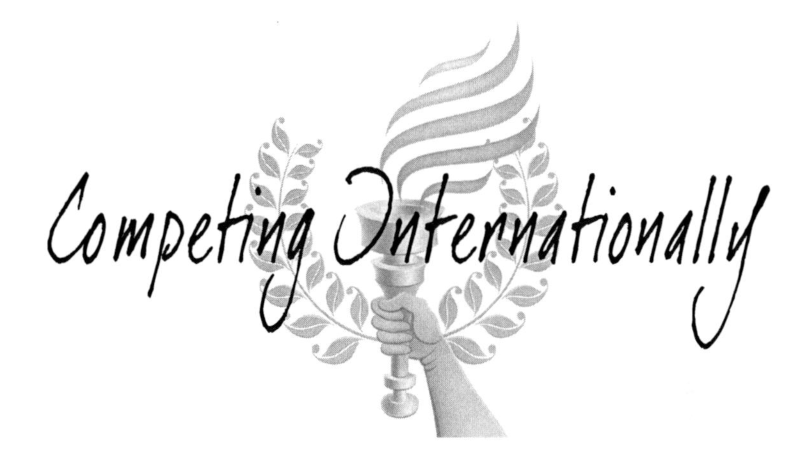

Some things never change, while others change constantly. Besides exhibitions, we spent our time after Nationals looking for new music and developing our 1982 routines. Because we placed well at Nationals, we qualified to be in the running for two international competitions, where we tested and fine-tuned our program.

Our first international competition was Skate Canada in Calgary. Even though I had competed in Canadian open competitions, traveling with an international team was totally different. As part of an invitation-only team, we got to hang out and make friends with the best of the best in the ice skating world. These were elite athletes we had watched from afar a few years earlier.

Peter, who also participated with us in the event, sat with me on the flight to Calgary, while Kitty sat with Lisa. As Peter was sizing up the competition for me, Lisa interrupted his analysis by popping up over the back of the seat in front of me.

"Scott!" she whispered.

I looked at her and almost laughed. She was ogling some of the ice skating celebs in the rows around us like a wide-eyed tourist. Then it hit me: I probably looked like one too.

"Yeah?"

"How are we going to compete with these people? I mean, these guys are, like, you know!"

I looked at Peter, and he started laughing, hard.

Kitty's head popped up beside Lisa's. "What's so funny?" she asked, ready to launch a sibling duel at fifteen thousand feet.

"Well?" Lisa demanded an answer.

"I suppose we'll do what we always do," I replied, the older, wiser, and more experienced one of our partnership. "We'll just do what we've been trained to do. Don't worry, we'll be all right."

"But, we've never competed internationally!" she said, her voice quavering. "What if we come in last? I'd be so embarrassed."

Her words hit the mark for a second.

"Relax," Peter interjected, with a grin on his face.

"That's easy for you to say," Lisa said.

"I've been trying to convince her that she'll be fine," Kitty said, glaring at her brother, almost daring him to make a smart remark.

"We won't come in last," I laughed nervously.

Kitty's glare whiplashed from her brother to me.

I quickly finished my remark. "We did well at Nationals with less than a year as partners, didn't we?"

Kitty returned her stare to Peter, who cleared his throat. "Yeah, well, um, it's natural to feel jittery your first time out. You'll be fine. You're not the only first-timers here, you know."

Lisa hesitated a moment. "I guess I'm just scared," she replied. "I feel like I'm so out of my league."

"I know what you mean," I said, "but isn't this what we've been working for?" Before she could respond, the flight attendant stopped and asked the girls to turn around so they could be served drinks and snacks.

Lisa's fears were quelled once we arrived and got into the rhythm of the competition. We finished in a respectable fourth place at Skate Canada and gained a foothold as a team to watch in the years ahead.

Our second international competition was in Holland, which is part of the Netherlands in western Europe, bordering the North Sea between Belgium and Germany. I loved the old-world feel of the country, despite the six-hour time difference that led to my first real experience with jet lag.

We did manage to get in some sightseeing. I was amazed by the way the cities interact with the water through their use of canal systems. Flooding is a real problem there, so they have developed sophisticated water management systems that enable them to use waterways, much like we use paved streets. Canal boats are used for mass transit, much like buses are in U. S. cities. The other primary mode of transportation is bicycling. It seems like every space there is carefully planned and used, which only makes sense with almost seventeen million people living in an area slightly less than the size of two New Jerseys.

Our huge hotel was located right on the water, which I thought was great. Even though the water's surface was more expansive than the lake in Skaneateles, it gave me a sense of home. Another lifestyle difference I noticed was that dogs often accompanied their owners into restaurants. Yeah, I really did like Holland.

Another awesome sight actually came from the competition itself—Natalia Bestemianova and her partner, Andrei Bukin, one of the top-ranked Russian teams. Natalia could twizzle so fast that you thought her head would fling off! Her mastery of the multirotational, one-foot turn was amazing.

We placed in the middle of the pack in Holland. Our evaluations in these international events gave us a good sense of how our programs played before the judges. Based on their response, we adjusted the programs in preparation for major competitions, especially the U. S. National Championships scheduled for Indianapolis that year.

Our second year together was just as exciting and intense as the first year, perhaps even more so because we were considered contenders. We weren't Luddy's only rising stars; he was quickly building his reputation for training champions.

Fast friendships formed among those of us who traveled on the international team. Major players like Scott Hamilton, David Santee, and Brian Boitano were among those whom we got to know. These U. S. and international champions were approachable and quick to accept us into the fold. Their warmth and encouragement made us feel as though we were part of something bigger.

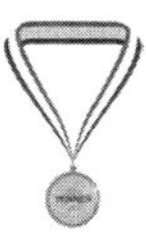

After placing well in the 1981 competition, Lisa and I were ready for Nationals. Our confidence in our skill level, combined with a rigorous training schedule, paid off during the competition. We came in third, which earned us a spot on the World team. Due to our adrenaline high from our win and our excitement over what lay ahead, we celebrated well into the wee hours of the morning.

Needless to say, my body wasn't happy when the front desk wake-up call pulled me out of bed early Sunday morning. With our World team meeting less than an hour away and an exhibition scheduled for the afternoon, I put my "getting-the-day-started" routine on autopilot. Despite my best efforts, I looked pretty ragged when I met Lisa in the lobby. She didn't look much better when we joined other World team members heading for the hotel's banquet rom.

A continental breakfast awaited us and our fellow champions in the meeting room. Where were the sharp athletes who earned their rankings as the best of the nation less than twelve hours earlier? They started emerging after their second cups of coffee. That's when the World team organizers came in to brief us on what to expect, and they didn't come empty-handed.

All of us skaters sat around the conference room tables while our coaches stood in the back of the room. Luddy, who looked quite pleased since four of his teams were going to the Worlds, stood in the back of the room with his arms folded in front of him. The officials spoke for twenty minutes about what to expect and how to conduct ourselves as the U. S. delegation during the March 9-14 Copenhagen competition. Then staff members passed out World team winter jackets, warm-up suits, skate bags, and a variety of sponsors' gifts that would be beneficial during the weeks ahead.

When I received my jacket, suddenly it hit me: everything was coming together. It was happening, just as I had dreamed it would.

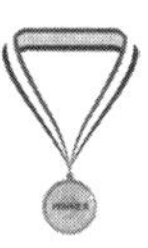

We rested for two days after we got home and then went back into competition mode by strengthening our programs for Copenhagen. The month went by quickly. It was truly a different experience for me, because my season usually never extended beyond Nationals. Preparing for the Worlds thrust me into two more months of intensive training. Having Peter, a seasoned World participant, as a housemate and best friend helped.

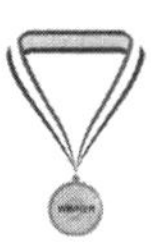

In Copenhagen, I was so focused on this huge international event that our location seemed like nothing more than a backdrop. For Lisa and me, the Worlds was a major paradigm shift. Experiencing competition at this extremely high level was our new reality, with all its particular perks and perils. Winning at this time seemed unattainable, like trying to climb a six-foot ladder by starting at the top rung. In other words, it was physically impossible. Climbing the ladder one or two rungs at a time could take us higher than we dared to dream.

After completing the registration ritual in Copenhagen and settling into our hotel rooms, we started our three-day regimen of eating, practice, and rest. Practice sessions were set up for six teams on the ice at the same time. We happened to be in the same practice group as Jayne Torvill and Christopher Dean, the reigning world champions from Great Britain, who had to be at least ten years ahead of their time.

Observing their conduct and how they trained helped us. Extremely businesslike and totally focused, they didn't engage in conversation with many people at all. They communicated with their coach, skated their programs, and then left.

It was hard to not feel self-conscious and inferior with them in the same room. They didn't see us, but we certainly saw them.

"Look at them," I said, as Lisa and I stood on the ice.

"Yeah," she sighed. "They're beyond awesome. They're . . ."

Reluctantly, I pulled my attention away from the perfect team and started to practice. When our session was over, we followed the greatest of the greats off the ice.

When our first three days ended, three days of competition began. Our order of performance was left to the luck of the draw, which actually put us skating right before Torvill and Dean in the first compulsory event—France was first, then Russia, followed by the U. S., and finally Great Britain. A total of twenty-two teams competed in the ice-dancing category. The digital scoreboard above the center of the ice kept the competitors' rankings in view for all to see. After the first compulsory dance, we ranked eighth, where we more or less remained for the entire competition. When the last team finished the last performance, it was official: We ranked eighth in the world.

We had climbed the first rung, which was not too shabby. Commentators were now touting Spitz and Gregory among the front-runners on the U. S. ice-dancing circuit. One of the greatest threats facing any competitor, however, is the possibility of becoming overconfident—thinking that he or she has arrived and there's clear sailing ahead.

My dad, a former fighter pilot who appreciated the value of discipline and training, closely scrutinized our training program, analyzed our progress, and felt compelled to offer advice that he believed would give us an edge in future competitions, which would ultimately take us to the 1984 Winter Olympics. That fall, he wrote the following letter, dated October 13, 1982.

Dear Scott,

There's no need for me to write, "My heart is heavy"—not at this time. Mom and I are so very proud of you.

The time seems to be fast approaching—the climb up the proverbial ladder . . . waiting your turn . . . it's almost here. It's ever so close. But as you know, you cannot rest. Just as you have now beaten those that were ahead of you, there are those below you waiting for you to err.

"Rosie Girl" (Lisa's mother) harps at you over and over, but in many respects she's correct. While Luddy is away (traveling with some other teams), you should plan on getting all the outside help you can. This should not be limited to skating but should also include dance, mime, choreography, and gymnastics. It may also be wise to start up again with the weights.

In spite of it all, you've done great! It just seems a little bit more could easily put you on top.

See you soon,
Dad

While I hadn't been keen on the extra-curricular activities, I saw the wisdom in my dad's advice and decided to accept the outside help instead of just tolerating the extras. Embracing it made this side of my training more fun. Since our ice time was so limited at the Skate Club of Wilmington, we opted to drive to Havertown, Pennsylvania, five days a week to get in a few more hours of practice. The new strategy was paying off, making the 1982-83 season our virtual golden years when we won Skate America and Skate Canada competitions. We were quite at home in first place, sometimes placing ahead of future Olympic medalists, and steadily climbing the ladder with higher placement in most events.

By the 1984 season, subtle changes started intruding into our relationship, creating a quiet but ever-growing tension between us. I don't think either of us noticed it in the beginning, but when we started slipping in the standings we knew then that something was wrong. Unfortunately, we avoided the issues rather than confronting them openly.

About a month before the 1984 Nationals, which was supposed to be our last push to make the Olympic team, things came to a head. Kitty and Lisa drove to Havertown in one car, while Peter and I drove up in another. We planned to go through our programs, regardless of glitches and errors. When competing, you can never quit if you do something wrong. Practicing despite the problems reinforces the mindset to continue, no matter what. Just like during our earliest days as partners, Lisa and I had different views on preparing to push through.

On that particular day, Lisa and Kitty had gone into the ladies' restroom together while Peter and I were on the ice warming up. About five minutes later, Kitty came out.

"Where's Lisa?" I asked, a bit impatient because the clock was ticking.

"She'll be out in a few minutes," Kitty said, joining her brother. As she walked away, I heard her finish her comment with a fading "I hope."

So I stood there waiting. I checked my watch, getting angrier as the sweep hand ticked away one more second.

"Come on, Lisa," I called out toward the closed door. "We've got to practice."

Silence greeted my growing anger. I couldn't believe Lisa's lack of consideration.

Pacing back and forth in front of the ladies' room, which was close to the boards, I waited another five minutes. I even considered entering this no man's land and pulling her out, but I knew that wouldn't do any good.

After their warm-ups, Peter and Kitty skated toward me. "What's up, Scott? Where's Lisa?" Peter asked.

"She still hasn't come out," I said, turning toward them.

"I'll go check on her," Kitty said, stepping off the ice and slipping on her blade guards.

"Don't bother," I said. "I'm done. I'm leaving."

"I'll come with you," Peter said as he started to follow his sister.

"No," I said. "You've paid for your ice time. Use it." I stuffed my gear in my bag and huffed out of the arena and into the parking lot.

Potential conversations and confrontations played through my mind during my drive back to Wilmington. I drove straight to the skating club and searched for Luddy. I found him sitting on a stool by the ice in teaching mode. I walked over to him and waited.

Luddy left me standing there for about forty-five seconds and finally turned his head toward me. "What's up?"

"I've had it, Luddy," I said.

He maneuvered the rest of his body to face me and gave me his full attention.

I vented as I told him what happened in Havertown, releasing the frustration that had been growing since the beginning of the year.

"Are you finished?" he asked after the words stopped tumbling from my mouth.

Here it comes, I thought. *He's going to blast me for leaving the way I did.*

"I think you need to get away for a few days."

"What?" That was the last thing I expected.

"Take a few days off, but don't tell anyone where you're going. I won't either. Let her sweat for a while."

I wasn't sure where this strategy would take me, but perhaps a cooling-off period would be good for both of us. So I went home, packed my bags, and headed home for Skaneateles.

I stayed home, getting more irritated that she hadn't figured out where I went. I spent most of my time hanging out with Don and venting about my Lisa issues. Because Don was such a good friend, he was a great outlet for my frustrations.

On the morning of the fourth day, the phone rang. Without thinking, I removed the receiver from its cradle.

"Scott?" Lisa's voice was wobbly.

"Yeah," I knew I sounded like a ten-year-old in the middle of a temper tantrum.

"I'm sorry," she said. I could tell that she was crying. I hate it when women cry because I'm never sure what to do with that.

"Sorry doesn't get us ready for Nationals," I groused.

"I know," she said. "I'm sorry I was such a brat. I'm willing to do whatever it takes to prepare. I promise."

I was back in Wilmington by early afternoon, and we were practicing that night. Despite winning the argument, thanks to Luddy, I sensed that things were starting to fall apart. Valuable time was lost, and I didn't like that feeling at all.

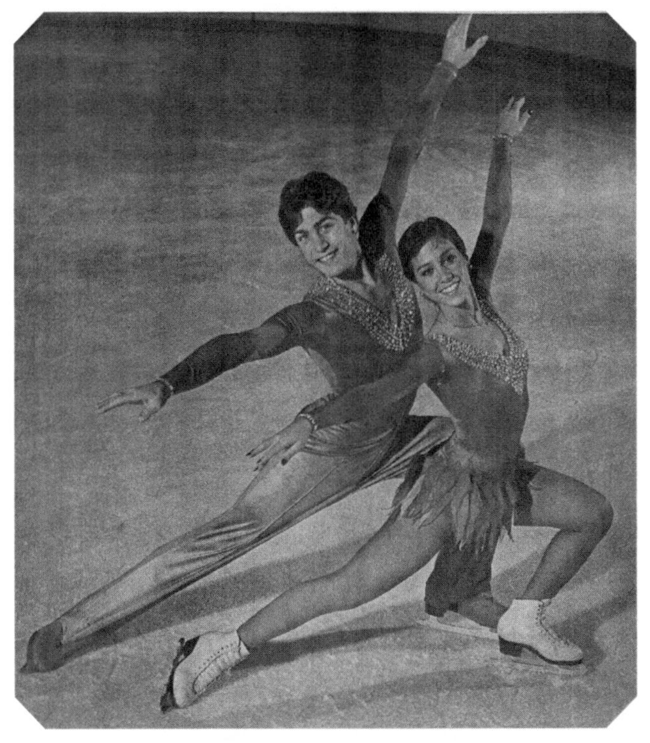

Lisa and I, putting our differences aside and getting down to business, preparing for Nationals in Salt Lake City.

Chapter 17

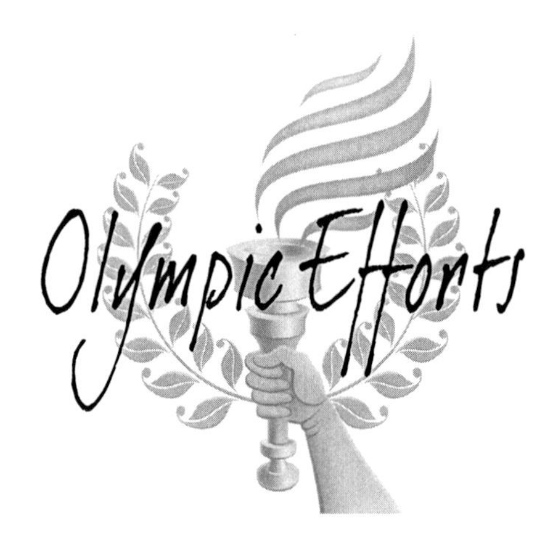

Olympic Efforts

True to her word, Lisa made it to the rest of our practices. We were generally cordial and friendly but didn't interact much in our free time. As a team, however, we were like an almost itch that may or may not need to be scratched. Even though we were reading the same book, we weren't necessarily on the same page.

When a team isn't operating in absolute unity, winning becomes difficult—if not nearly impossible. Unity is the thread that holds it all together, but discord tears it apart.

Nationals were in Salt Lake City that year. If I wasn't aware of our growing differences before the Havertown stand-off, our performance in Salt Lake should have tipped me off. Our home-rink rivals, Carol Fox and Richard Dalley, edged us into a third-place position, while they sailed right into second. Since we were second the year before, I anticipated at least the same in 1984. But we qualified for the Olympics, and that's what counted. Less than a week after we returned home, I received a letter from my mother:

January 28, 1984

Dear Scott,

I wish we could express to you how proud we are as parents to have a child who has worked so hard for so many years with such complete devotion for a desire and goal such as you have, and made it. To think that you've worked so long for this day, and now it is here and you did it.

I always knew way back in the day when we watched you in Rochester that you had the talent and personality to someday make it to the Olympics if you only had the true desire. The Edmunds and Syracuse crowd always told me you would make it, and we believed them too. There were certainly some ups and downs, and sometimes we thought you weren't going to stick it out. But you did, and we are so proud, thrilled, excited, and stunned to believe that it's all come true. I hope it was something you really wanted, and you didn't do it just for us. I hope we didn't seem pushy at times—if we did, we only wanted to encourage you, for we knew you were exceptional.

You and Lisa give much joy, pleasure, and inspiration to those who know and watch you. We want to thank you for the sacrifices you have made to achieve this high and unique honor. Everyone who knows you is so proud of you.

Something so precious about it all is that you are the same Scott you were since day one. Your personality and unselfish ways have not been changed by all the glamour, and this is such a precious asset. We know it would not have been worth it if you had changed and become a snob and know-it-all.

How blessed we were to have such a wonderful son and another wonderful son and daughter, to boot. They were so great not to demand more of our time, which would have taken away from your training.

May the Lord watch over you and bless you in these trying, difficult, and exciting days ahead. We will be praying that you both will skate your very best and feel the best about your skating. This is all one can do—to satisfy one's self.

Much love,
Mom & Dad

Mom's letter encouraged me to believe in myself and my dreams. It came at a good time, motivating me to overcome the bumps ahead. There was little time to dwell on our differences, though, because we were one of four teams from Luddy's stable going to the Olympics. This stirred a minor media frenzy during our two months of preparation. What little local celebrity we might have enjoyed catapulted us to national and international attention. Yet we took it all in stride, focusing instead on our preparation.

But the increased attention and positive tension didn't seem to help Lisa and me. We kept running hot and cold, in our professional relationship and training. Communication is a key component of unity, but Lisa and I were barely talking to each other. Even riding the cusp of the media attention wave wasn't enough to keep us going. Since we weren't always on the same page, my frustration level rapidly increased. Peter helped keep me on track, but that wasn't enough either. It didn't take long for Luddy to speak up.

Ten minutes into our session that week after we returned from Salt Lake, Luddy motioned us over to his rink-side stool. Lisa and I half-glared at each other and then back to Luddy.

"Is there a problem here?" Luddy asked quietly.

"No, no problem," I replied softly.

"Yeah," Lisa replied. "We're good to go."

"You're not acting like it," he said, sharply. "Come on, guys, get it together. Get along, and get the work done!"

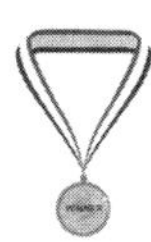

The Olympics is everybody's dream and one of the final mountains to climb. This international event is the point of great achievement that demonstrates excellence at its best. Luddy's admonishment helped to refocus us on the dream. Soon, we were days away from leaving for Sarajevo in the Socialst Federal Republic of Yugoslavia. Our excitement seemed to smooth out our differences, allowing us to realize that we were part of something much bigger than we'd ever experienced before in our lives.

Finally, Luddy's four teams and our assistant coach, Robbie Kaine, were at the Philadelphia International Airport dressed in our "Team USA" jackets, responding to questions from the regional press and posing for pictures of us holding a large Olympic flag.

Seated on the airplane next to Peter, I heard the engines roaring at take-off.

"Scott, listen to this," Peter said as he gave me the earphones to his Walkman. Rush with Getty Lee, a Canadian group, was singing "Take Off to the Great White North."

As the comedic song ended, he said, "Next stop, Sarajevo."

Peter always knew how to make me laugh. The two of us started laughing almost uncontrollably.

Kitty poked her head around the corner of the aisle seat. "What's so funny?"

"Nothing," Peter replied, as we both grinned.

"What?" Kitty said, teasing irritation hugging the edge of her voice.

"All right," Peter said, still laughing. "Listen to this." He handed the Walkman to his sister. A few minutes later, we heard giggles from the seat in front of us. We were off to a good start.

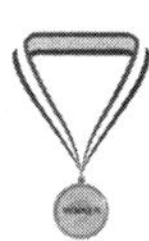

Once we landed in Sarajevo, we went to the Olympic Village. After enduring multiple security checkpoints, Peter, Kitty, Lisa, and I entered into a wonderland filled with athletes from every part of the globe standing in various lines. A volunteer ushered us to the registration table. We each picked up an identification badge and various passes. As our ushers led us to a line of shopping carts, I looked at Peter, who just grinned.

"Shopping carts?" I asked. "That's a first."

"Not really," Peter said, as he selected a cart and got in line. Doing the same, I followed him.

We started at the U. S. A. section, where we each received our opening ceremonies outfit—a cowboy hat, a camel-skin coat, gloves, lined Levi blue jeans, boots, and gloves. I was beginning to understand our need for the carts. We went to additional stations for a sports jacket, khaki pants, shirt, tie, long underwear, ski jackets, bibbed ski pants, winter hat, belt and buckle with the Olympic emblem, and Olympic ring and watch, along with a suitcase to carry everything back home. Everything we received had the Olympic logo and year embroidered or attached to it.

After a few days of practice and acclimating ourselves to the European winter, it was time for the opening ceremonies. I can't begin to describe how participating in that incredibly powerful event affected me. It was enough to give me chills.

The U. S. flag came out of the tunnel, followed by the American team dressed in full western gear, including cowboy hats. With the girls in the front of the line and the guys in the back, Kitty and Lisa were among the first to enter. Scott Hamilton and I were in the first row of the men. Almost in unison, we took our hats off and waved at the crowd. People in the stands cheered, many of them standing to their feet and waving American flags. It was unbelievable. The roar of the crowd was uplifting. With this kind of intense enthusiasm, who wouldn't want to do their best in this environment?

To be a part of this made all the tears, injuries, and hard work worth it. My heart overflowed, and my mind raced. *This is the one event in your athletic career that you've prepared for all your life, whether you realized it in the early years or not. Doing well is not optional, but mandatory, especially with the added pressure of being viewed all over the world—there are no higher stakes.*

I was happy with our performance during the ten-day event. With the exception of one compulsory dance during which we had a slight glitch that didn't affect the routine, we had never skated better together. But every flaw counts, so we came in tenth. I found our placement disappointing and lower than I had hoped.

Despite my disappointment, nothing could tarnish the extraordinary experience of participating in the Olympics. Our next stop was the Worlds in Ottawa in March.

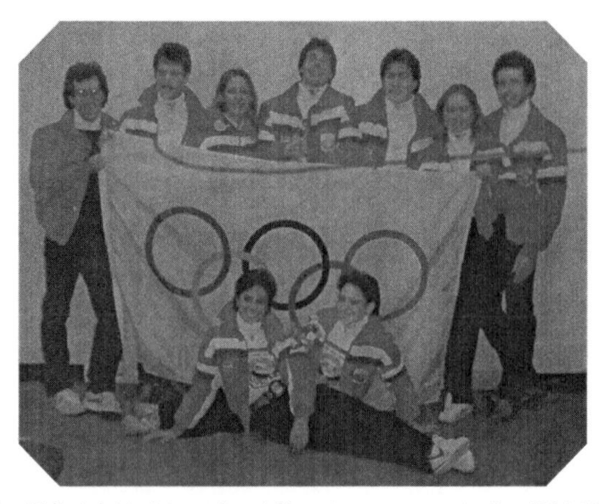

The USA team at the Philadelphia International Airport, on our way to the 1984 Olympics in Sarajevo, Yugoslavia. Left to right (standing): Coach Robbie Kane, Richard Deally, Carol Fox, Peter Carruthers, me, LeAnn Miller, Bill Fauver; (sitting) Lisa Spitz, and Kitty Carruthers. Psyched, ready to get there!

Chapter 18

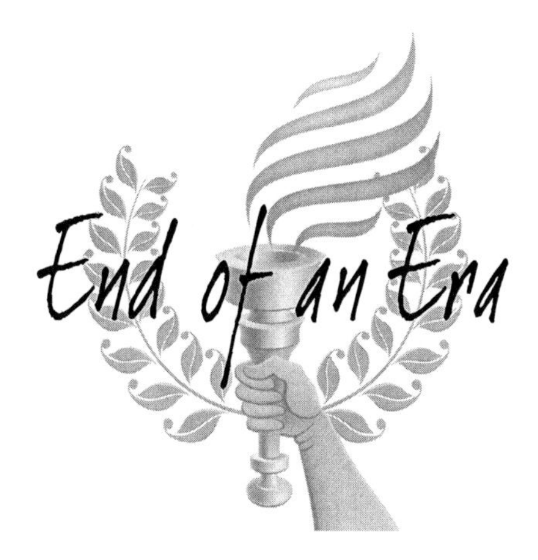

End of an Era

When we returned to Wilmington, we settled back into our old routine. With four more events (one competition and three exhibitions) to complete before the end of the season, we continued in training mode until the Worlds in March. While we were still on the Olympic high, things were great; but within a week or so, it was obvious that Lisa was dissatisfied, because she was yearning for a normal life. We were hot and cold with a "let's go in and get our work done so we can go our separate ways," overtone tainting everything we did. Our focus was on keeping ourselves in shape, while our training was on autopilot. Even so, nothing could dampen my anticipation for our first exhibition in my hometown, which was scheduled for a few weeks before the Worlds.

We were doing my hometown show because of a telegram I received while we were in Sarajevo. Skaneateles municipal officials congratulated me on competing in the Olympics and proclaimed March 3 as Scott

Gregory Day. Since Peter and Kitty were silver medalists and our best friends, we asked them to join us in the exhibition on "my" day.

Instead of driving up, we flew into Syracuse on the Thursday before the exhibition. After we arrived at the airport and started looking for my mom's familiar face, I started growing a little concerned when I didn't see her, until Peter noticed a man in a chauffeur's uniform with a "Scott Gregory" sign standing at the baggage claim exit. What a surprise, returning home in style!

The limousine was quite a change from buses and coach seating. We enjoyed every minute of the forty-minute ride to Skaneateles, even the perfectly chilled champagne waiting for us. But instead of taking us to my parents' house, our trip ended at the Skaneateles Figure Skating Club for an informal reception.

I looked around the freshly painted lobby and snack area, where friends, family, and skating club members congregated to welcome home the conquering hero and his friends. It was hard to believe that this was the same open-air rink where I mastered the move "shoot the duck" during my eight-week trial thirteen years earlier. Building around the original structure, the skating rink now had a lobby, snack bar, and locker rooms. When Don, who was now a chef, wheeled in an ice sculpture and a cake, everyone applauded. It was one he had carved to commemorate the occasion.

Afterward, we went home with my parents, where the six of us sat around the kitchen table talking. "So, what will you and Kitty be doing, now that you have your medals?" my dad asked.

"We're turning pro," Peter said.

"Oh?" Dad looked really interested.

"We just signed with an agent," Peter continued. "He's from IMG."

"We're joining the Ice Capades," Kitty popped in. "It's exciting."

"We also have some decent endorsement deals to consider," Peter said, leaning back in his chair.

"It sounds like you're set," Dad said. Then he turned his attention to me. "So I guess you'll be looking for a new roommate soon."

"Too soon," I replied. "Peter's been a good friend. I'm going to miss him."

A big, fat tear trickled down Lisa's face. "I didn't think saying goodbye would be so hard," she said, her voice quite raspy.

I looked at her, somewhat startled.

"Scott did mention that you were planning to go to college this fall," Mom said.

Lisa nodded her head, her conflicting emotions reflected in her facial expressions.

Mom sat down next to Lisa and put her arms around her. "You and Scott have been good together. I'm glad you had these four years."

Looking at Mom with this petite girl who brought me so much frustration yet who stuck it out made me realize that she had made sacrifices too. I knew that she had, but seeing her here like this gave me a higher respect for her. A lot of people would have walked out as soon as they had the Olympics under their belts, but not Lisa. She was finishing the season. For the first time, I felt relaxed about her decision.

She looked up at me, more tears spilling onto her cheeks. I smiled at her and said "Yeah, me too."

Then the dam broke. Lisa started seriously crying now. My dad started laughing. "This is a celebration," he said, "not a time for tears." We sat in the kitchen for another two hours, revisiting events from the past four years and considering the different paths ahead.

On Friday afternoon, we participated in a parade that took us to the rink for the afternoon's exhibition. We wore our Olympic jackets to ward off the edge of winter's chill. Through overcast skies, the sun's warming rays hinted at the promise of spring. I saw Mom standing with friends and family in front of Dad's insurance agency, but Dad was conspicuously absent. Suddenly four A-37 fighter jets flew overhead. I started laughing.

"What's so funny?" Peter asked over the scream of the jet engines flying five hundred feet above the ground.

I pointed skyward, but Peter still looked puzzled.

"That's my dad and his Air Guard pals," I shouted back.

Peter looked up and started laughing with me. "That's awesome!"

Dad, his close friends Woody and Homer, and another pilot from Hancock Field Air National Guard Base in Syracuse, had just taken our parade to a higher level.

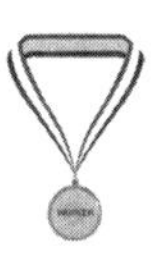

That evening we attended a testimonial dinner at the Sherwood Inn, a stagecoach stop back in 1807. Its rustic appearance and charm, along with its location in the heart of the lake's north shore, makes it one of the nicer places to dine in town.

Lisa, Kitty, and Peter were made honorary citizens of Skaneateles and received plaques designating their new position. I received a key to the city, along with something I'd always wanted—a blue high school letter jacket with a gold letter. Since figure skating was not a sanctioned high school sport, I didn't qualify for a sports jacket, but I guess the Olympics changed that.

I felt honored by the attention and the accolades. I was the town's first Olympian, so I supposed they had earned bragging rights.

Then it was time to wrap things up. Lisa, Kitty, and Peter left the next day, but I wanted to spend a few days at home before returning to our training.

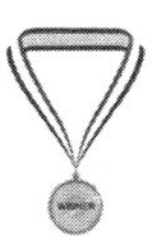

On Monday night, Don and I went to a local sports bar for dinner when someone from my past entered the dimly lit room. I tried to stifle a groan when a stocky man with scraggly blond hair stepped into the light.

"What's wrong?" Don asked.

"Oh, man," I muttered.

Don looked at me.

"I just saw someone I really don't want to talk to," I said. Suddenly, I felt like I was back at my locker at middle school.

"Who?" Don looked around. "Is it someone I know?"

"No," I said, feeling silly. "It's a guy who harassed me mercilessly in middle school."

Before I could explain, Butch spotted me.

"Hey, Scott!" he yelled across the room.

I tried to take a deep breath and suck it up. This was not how I planned to spend my last night in town. Within seconds, he was at our table.

"It's great to see you, man." He shook my hand as if I were his long-lost best buddy. I was speechless. "I saw you on television skating at the Olympics! Everyone's talking about you."

Before I could say thank you and good-bye, Butch sat down and started talking up a storm. He finally left when the waitress brought our meals.

"So," Don said after the waitress left. "This guy gave you some trouble back in the day."

"Go figure," I said as I looked up and saw him talking to some other fellows and pointing our way. "He used to make fun of me because I was a figure skater instead of a hockey player like he was. Now he acts like my best friend." I felt like I was in a fish bowl, but I suppose I would rather be on his good side than his bad.

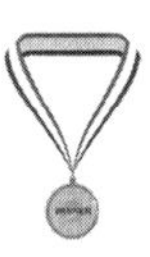

I returned to Wilmington on Tuesday to resume training with Lisa for the Worlds, a real letdown after our Olympics experience. Trying to continue our friendship with our "business-in-and-out" approach was a bit daunting, however. With Peter gone most of the time, I needed to find ways to keep motivated. The music from *Footloose*, a movie which was released a month earlier, was a big help at times. The music was so catchy and upbeat that I often found myself dancing around the house on 1430 Foulk Road like Gene Kelly dancing around on couches, chairs, and walls as props. At least this gave me some kind of outlet.

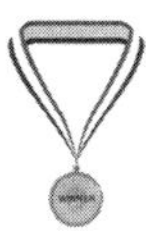

The Worlds in Ottawa proved to be more bitter than sweet for Lisa and me. Our last event, the free dance scheduled for 5 p.m., summed up the whole experience. I was mentally prepared to nail this number and move higher up in our standings. As part of the last group of six, we were just about to take the ice for our warm-ups when the fire alarm sounded. Subsequently, everyone was forced to leave the building. As we grabbed our gear and started walking outside, I noticed smoke coming from an area behind the stage, so it wasn't a false alarm.

Evacuating the rink meant returning to the hotel, putting on our street clothes, and waiting for the call to return. One hour drifted into two, three, and then four. While my fellow skaters were relaxing and enjoying the evening, Lisa and I were getting antsy and anxious.

"Man, this really stinks for you," Scott Hamilton said sincerely and teasingly at the same time. Of course, he was one to talk because he had already skated and won his event.

"You don't have to rub it in," I replied, trying to keep my mood light but disliking the emotional imbalance that was brewing within me. Finally, five hours after they sent us away, the officials called for the remaining competitors to return.

We didn't get back onto the ice until 11:30, and the competition finally closed about 1:30. We came in tenth, just like the Olympics. I was moving backwards in my standings, and I didn't like it.

Our flight back to Wilmington was strained. Lisa thought I was mad at her, but I wasn't.

"You understand, don't you, Scott?" Lisa's concern was genuine, but I didn't really want to talk about the end of our partnership or anything else.

"Don't shut me out, Scott." Her voice warbled as she started to cry. This was just what I needed on the plane ride back to the States.

"Yeah," I muttered, staring out the aircraft window. The inky sky showed through the small porthole, which reflected my own image with Lisa's head visible over my shoulder. "I understand."

But I didn't. We'd placed miserably both at the Olympics and the Worlds that year and now I had to go through the arduous task of finding some other partner if I wanted to continue. Only twenty-four, I felt worn down by the daunting task that lay ahead. Yet, after finally coming to terms with Lisa's decision, I was actually looking forward to getting a new partner.

"Scott, why won't you talk to me? I thought we, well, that—"

"Lisa, I'm not upset with you. I just can't believe we came in tenth when last year we were seventh. I'm going backwards!"

"Oh, that," she muttered. "Scott, it's over. You can't go back and redo it. Getting mad won't change the outcome. It's not that important."

"To you, maybe, but not for me."

Lisa shook her head, sighed, and tilted her seat back. She closed her eyes and was soon breathing the soft, rhythmic sighs of a sound sleeper. I continued to stare miserably out the window, facing the task ahead with mixed feelings.

"Now I have to start the whole thing all over again," I said softly to my reflected image. "So, where do I begin, and how much time will it cost me before the next competition? Will I make the World team? I want to and I have to, but I can't do it by myself. Who out there is ready to be my partner?"

I leaned my own seat back, hoping I'd have some answers by the time we had landed.

Shortly after our return, Lisa's hometown celebrated her successes much like Skaneateles did mine. In short order, we were headed for Salt Lake City, Utah, for our final exhibition together.

By that time I had shaken off our Worlds performance and focused on what was ahead. Knowing that this would be my last time with Lisa, all the frustration and aggravation melted away as we skated to our show number—a slow, strong, powerful, beautiful piece of music. By the time the last strains flowed throughout the arena, we both had some tears. For us, it was the end of an era.

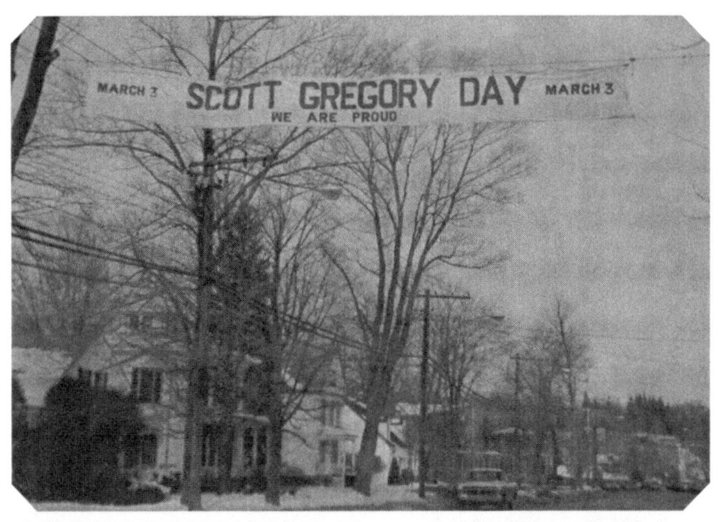

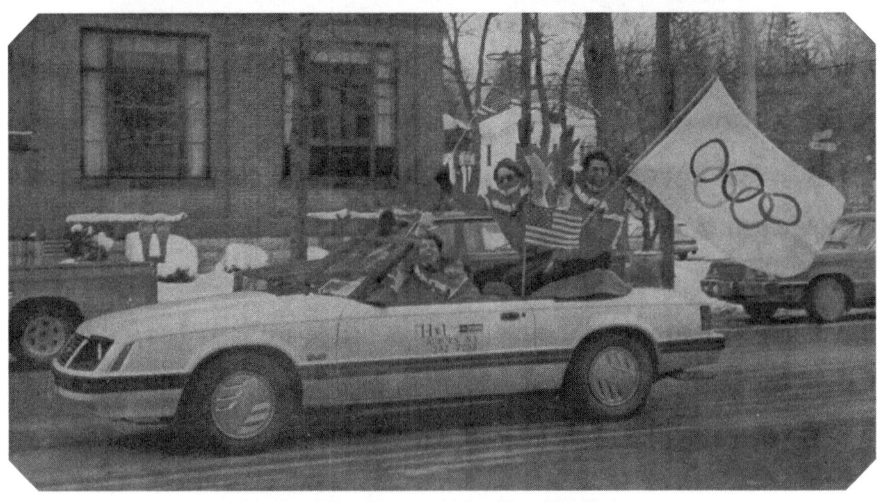

My friend Don Matson driving Lisa, Kitty, Peter,
and me in the *Scott Gregory Day* parade, March 3, 1984

Chapter 19

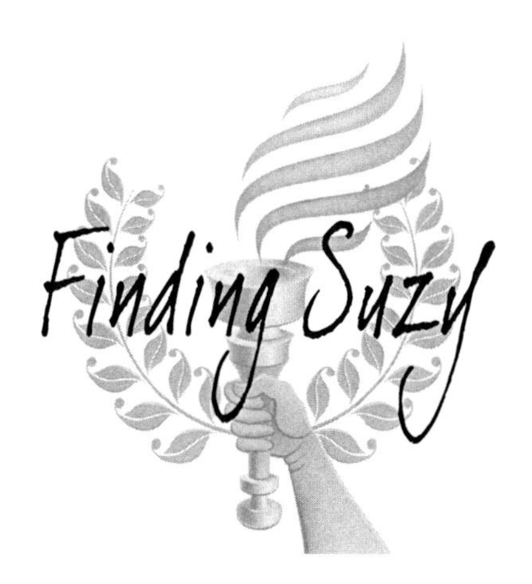

Finding Suzy

"Luddy?" I tentatively knocked on his office door. "Come in," he said, pushing aside the files in front of him. "Sit down."

Two steps into his office, I dropped my skate bag and sat in the closest chair. "You've heard?"

"Of course," he said, unabashed by the news. "When is she leaving?"

"She's already gone," I replied. "I'm not looking forward to starting over again with a new partner."

"What do you mean?"

"Finding someone else isn't going to be easy. I've put in my time. Now that it's my turn, Lisa up and leaves. I've got to start all over again! It just doesn't seem fair."

Luddy reached over and pulled a folder from the top of his stack of files. "You need someone strong," he said.

"What do you mean?"

"Scott, you're a seasoned competitor and an Olympian," he said, somewhat impatiently. "You're not the green kid who came in here four years ago!"

I shrugged my shoulders. "I suppose," I muttered, feeling as much adrift as I had when Judy left.

"Do you know what you're looking for in a new partner?" he asked curtly. "Have you developed a short list?"

"No and no," I replied.

"Well, you'd better figure it out soon because a coach from Pittsburgh just called." Luddy leaned forward, elbows on his desk.

"Really? And?"

"She has someone she thinks would be well worth your while to audition."

"Who?"

"Suzy Semanick," Luddy said, sliding the manila folder over to me. As I opened the file, I noticed her picture and qualifications. She was last year's junior national champion. Then I saw her age, laughed, and then groaned.

"What's the matter?"

"She's sixteen," I said. "Judy and Lisa were both sixteen when we started."

"Your point?" Luddy seemed as impatient as I felt.

"I'm twenty-four," I said. "I'm tired of breaking in kids."

"I understand," he said, "but you're getting good at it. She's expecting you in Pittsburgh in the next couple of days. Here's her phone number. Why don't you call her?"

"Could you come with me?"

"I can't," Luddy said. "Call Robbie. See if he'll go."

I drove back to the house and called Suzy to arrange a try-out. I had seen her earlier in the year when she came to the Skating Club of Wilmington to audition with a local skater. Luddy had me stroke with her a bit to demonstrate what he wanted her to do, and she picked it up fast. Her movements were also strong and aggressive.

Next, I called Robbie, who was willing and eager to help me find a new partner. I almost knew that Suzy was going to work out, and Robbie's viewpoint would either confirm or deny my expectations. We met at the Philadelphia airport two days later at 1 p. m. and flew to Pittsburgh.

"What are you thinking about, Scott?" Robbie slipped the airline magazine back into its pocket.

"About Suzy Semanick," I replied. "What do you think?"

Robbie laughed. "Well, she is the junior national champion, just like you were."

"Yeah, and look at what I had to go through to get better!"

"And you still have a ways to go to become your best," Robbie reminded me. "You know where you need to improve. Make a list of your strengths and weaknesses and how you want to be better. Then you can find someone who you think will be appropriate. Don't forget that even though it's going to be someone who wants to skate with you, it's not a one-way street. You have to be respectful of these young ladies."

"I try," I said, feeling as though a heavy weight was resting on my shoulders. "I hope my new partner wants this as badly as I do."

Moments later, the wheels were touching down on the tarmac. Suzy and her mom met us at the airport and drove us to the Mt. Lebanon recreational facility. Once there, we changed clothes and started warming up. I geared up and was on the ice a few moments later, but I couldn't see Suzy. Instead, a gaggle of twelve or so skaters were congregating near the far side of the rink. As I started skating toward them, I saw them whispering to one another.

"There he is!"

"He's really here."

A tall, dark-haired man broke ranks first.

"Hello," he said, skating toward me, right hand outstretched. "It's really an honor to meet you."

"Thanks," I replied, taking his hand.

A short, red-haired woman followed. "When we heard you were coming to skate with Suzy, we couldn't believe it," she said, giggling as she finished her greeting. "We saw you on television at the Olympics. You really should have placed much higher in the—"

"Scott!" Suzy skated in behind Red. "I would like to introduce you to some of my friends."

"Shall we skate?" I asked, after meeting her fellow skaters. Taking her other hand and circling the rink's exterior, I felt like we had been skating together for some time. After one pass around the rink, we skated over to Robbie. Much to my surprise, her friends melted into the sidelines to watch.

"I didn't know we'd have an audience," I muttered as we came to a halt in front of Robbie.

"Okay, you're looking good," Robbie said. "For your first couple of passes, do some stroking exercises. Then I want to see you do some basic dances."

Suzy seemed full of nervous energy, like a horse straining at the gate.

"That works for me," I said, taking her hand. "How about you?"

She nodded her head.

About two hours later, I noticed my brother, Bee Gee, standing by Robbie.

"Did you know my brother lives in Pittsburgh?" I asked Suzy after we finished one of the dances.

"No," she said.

"Yeah. That's him, over by Robbie. Can you stop by his house around six o'clock, after dinner?"

"Uh, sure," she replied, looking slightly bashful.

"I just need to ask you a few questions to make sure we're on the same page."

"Okay," she said.

We skated over to Robbie so she could meet Bee Gee and get his address, and then we parted. Suzy headed for the women's locker room, and I went to the men's. As I was leaving, school-age skaters started arriving. I started walking toward Robbie and Bee Gee when a tall girl who looked like she was about ten years old stopped me.

"You're Scott Gregory," she said quite matter-of-factly.

"Yes, I am." I was surprised by her recognition.

"I saw you skate in the Olympics." I wondered if she was related to Red. Her light brown hair did have some red highlights.

"Yeah?" I replied, unsure of the direction of this conversation.

"How did you do it?"

"What?"

"How did you get to the Olympics?"

I thought for a minute. How did I get there? "I started when I was about your age," I said rather tentatively. "Well, it's a lot of hard work, and you can't quit—no matter what."

She stood there for a moment. "Thanks," she said. "I'll remember that." Then she turned and half-skipped away.

Moments later, I joined Robbie and Bee Gee at rink-side. "So, what do you think?"

"You look good together," Robbie said.

"She's the one," I replied, trying to hold down my enthusiasm. "I just know it."

Bee Gee and I drove Robbie back to the airport and then headed to my brother's house in the suburbs of Pittsburgh. We had just finished clearing the dinner dishes from the table when the doorbell rang. Moments later, we were sitting in the living room, plying Suzy with questions. By the end of our conversation, I concluded that she was way too serious.

"Well, you are clearly a good skater, sincere and dedicated," I said, equally serious. "And you've answered all my questions. Now, let's see how daring you are. Get up and dance on the table."

Suzy stared at me, puzzled, like a doe in front of the headlights. "Dance?"

"Yeah, come on," I continued, barely able to control my voice. Bee Gee got it, but his wife, Sharon, stared at me like I'd lost my mind. Suzy looked like she was totally scared, but she started to step up onto the table.

"Scott!" Sharon shouted as I started laughing. She sounded more like my mom than my sister-in-law.

"Just kidding," I said sheepishly before Suzy climbed up all the way. Bee Gee burst into fits of laughter. Neither Sharon nor Suzy seemed to appreciate my little joke.

"We have to meet with Luddy when we get back, but I'm sure he'll be calling your coach tomorrow."

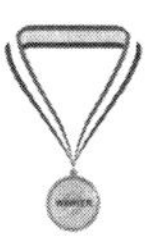

Our mission accomplished, I took an early flight back to Philadelphia the next morning. I had found Suzy, so I was ready to start all over again. And this time, I just knew it would work out well—it just *had* to.

Having been on the World team the last three years, I wanted to be right back on top my first year with Suzy. I hoped she wanted the same.

Chapter 20

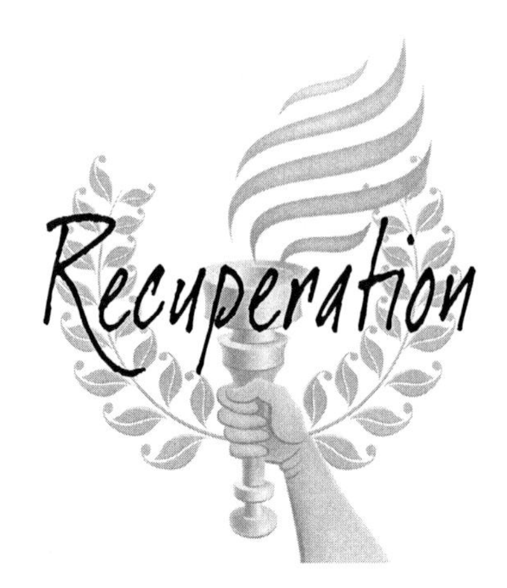

Recuperation

On the way home from the airport, I stopped by the rink to report to Luddy, but I was too late. He had received a full update from Robbie before I even got back.

"That didn't take long," he said, leaning back in his chair, his hands interlaced behind his head.

"Yeah," I leaned forward, chuckling. I was far more relaxed than the last time I was in his office.

"What's next?"

"I'll call Suzy tonight and tell her to come to Wilmington."

Luddy smiled. "That sounds like a plan," he said. Then he changed the subject to a topic I wished to avoid. "What about your surgery?"

During the last two years, I had experienced an annoyingly noticeable pain that didn't stop me from skating, but it certainly didn't help. The doctors told me that the screw holding my kneecap together was the source of my discomfort.

"I hate to miss this time," I said, sighing.

"Better now than later," Luddy said. "We'll get Suzy broken in. It's your job to recuperate before we start our new season." The phone rang, pulling his attention to the next problem in his busy day. I quietly slipped out of the office and met some friends in the snack bar before I went home.

With Suzy settled in and her training schedule started, I felt better about taking the next four weeks off. Back in Skaneateles recuperating from surgery, I was remarkably refreshed. It was one of the few times in four years that I wasn't in training.

My first week home, I had two visitors—Lisa and one of my housemates, Todd Wagner. He was a pairs skater who had moved in about a year and a half before Peter left. With Peter gone, we naturally became closer friends.

Fortunately, my crutches didn't slow me down too much. The weather was picture perfect the whole time. We went out on my dad's twenty-three foot 1966 Century mahogany wood boat with a 280-horsepower Chrysler engine. It had a lot of power, which was particularly enjoyable in my current recuperative condition. The engine sang with its own unique voice as I opened up the throttle. The thrust and movement reminded me of the times as a child when the wind carried me along the ice with my makeshift sails.

I loved that boat with its wood-varnished siding, sliding top, and white stripe up the side. Being out on the lake with the boat drove away all my lingering doubts about skating and starting over. Of course, that's when Lisa popped the question.

"I hear you found a new partner."

Her fingers tickled the water alongside the boat.

"Yeah," I said softly, unsure of where this was all going.

"Is she any good?"

"Yeah," I replied, cautiously.

"Better than I am?"

How do you answer that question? "Different," I replied, "but on equal footing."

"Good." Lisa looked up at me for the first time during the conversation. "You deserve another shot."

I looked at Lisa, who would always be an incredibly good friend. Suddenly, any remnants of anger and frustration toward her disappeared. She *was* a good friend. We had accomplished remarkable things together—things that would never be taken away.

"Thanks," I said. "That means a lot. When do you start school?"

"In two months. It's different, not spending all my time at the rink, but it's a good thing too."

"Yeah," I said. "But I don't know if I could stand to stay away forever."

"That's the difference between us," she said.

I had to chuckle. "I suppose it is."

On the night after Lisa left, I called to check on Suzy. When I called her at the rink, I was almost surprised to reach her.

"Scott, this is fantastic!" Suzy's voice practically vibrated over the phone lines.

"Yeah."

"When will you be back?"

"In a week," I replied.

"Great!" she said. "I can't wait to start skating with you. It's going to be great!" A sound from behind seemed to distract her for a moment. "They're calling for me! Can you believe it? It's awesome, all the big-name skaters who are here. See you in a few!"

Before I could respond, the receiver went dead. "Great," I chuckled, mildly amused at this feeling of being on the outside looking in. I hated to see my time at home end, but I also wanted to get back on the ice.

Todd stayed in Skaneateles another week so he could drive me back to Wilmington. Even with Todd there, I managed to spend some time around the lake by myself. I hadn't realized how much I had been pushing myself through the years. During this time off, I seemed to cram a whole summer vacation into my two weeks at home.

All too soon, it was time to return. Todd and I were scheduled to drive back to Wilmington the next morning, so I decided to take Dad's boat out on the lake one last time.

The weather that day was perfect, so halfway out in the lake I turned off the engine, laid back in the seat, propped my feet up, and put my hands behind my head. The sun's heat was tempered by the lakefront breeze. Fresh water gently slapping against the side of the boat lulled me into a dream state. Thoughts of the past washed over me.

You've come a long way, Scott, I heard a small voice whisper inside my head.

"Yeah," I replied, "a long way since I sneaked my dad's skates out of the closet. But I could have gone a lot farther if I'd never been injured."

Things happen for a reason, the voice replied.

I started following the cryptic thought stream. "What if my injuries aren't punishment?" I said softly, just beginning to embrace the notion. "I mean, what's talent? My talent isn't who I am. I'm still Scott, whether I skate great or not. But, if I hadn't had these injuries, I would probably rely too heavily on my talent and neglect perseverance." My thoughts drifted into silence. Suddenly, I felt a warmth flow throughout my body, a healing touch that seemed to wash away frustration, disappointment, and all the emotional baggage that was holding me back.

"Whoa," I said as the sensation dissipated. The sun was starting to set. "Gee, it was almost like God was talking to me." I shook my head, thinking that a God-encounter was highly unlikely, but still, that cryptic voice was pretty convincing.

I looked around the lakeside, up the hills to the farmlands, and down to the north of the lake, where the village of Skaneatales reflected against the peaceful waters. I noticed a glow settling around the Episcopalian church, the house of worship I attended when I was a little boy. "Of course it was God," I muttered. It was too powerful to be anything else. As I settled into certainty, I felt a warmth that seemed to radiate His approval.

I wasn't sure how long I'd been on the lake, but it was certainly the better part of the afternoon. As I started the engine and headed toward shore, my thoughts lingered on the encounter. Grasping its meaning, I realized that by getting in touch with my spiritual side, God was with me even when I was too busy to notice.

Suddenly, the little things that drove me nuts were no longer important. I now had a bigger picture and a broader perspective. When I realized that He was on my side, I knew then that I could do anything. I had a strong sense that the next four years would be awesome. I knew that I was ready to go back and get started. I was excited.

Two days later, I was back at the rink, two weeks after the summer program began. My leg was stiff and my knee weak. I felt like a runner who almost ran the race but fell down before dashing across the finish line. The incisions on my knee were three inches long and not fully healed. But with each session, my leg strengthened and the stiffness diminished. It took stubborn strength to push past my stiffness and keep up with Suzy, but I relied on my new commitment to persevere. Before long, I was up to speed.

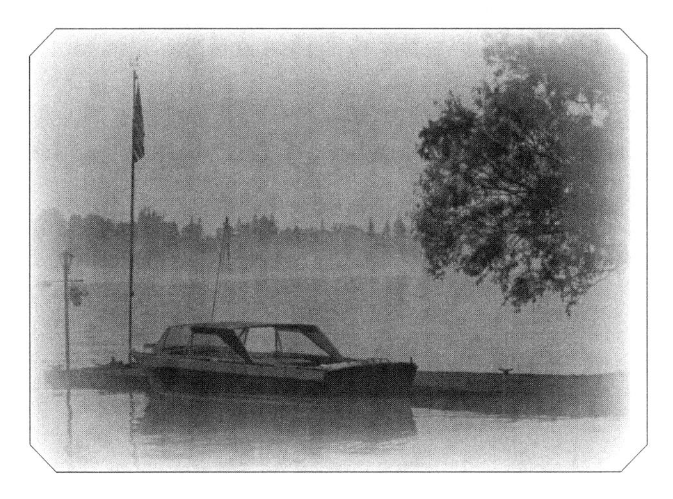

I call this "God's country," as shown from my back yard.
My dad's wooden boat on Skaneateles Lake became my sanctuary in the mid-1980s.

Chapter 21

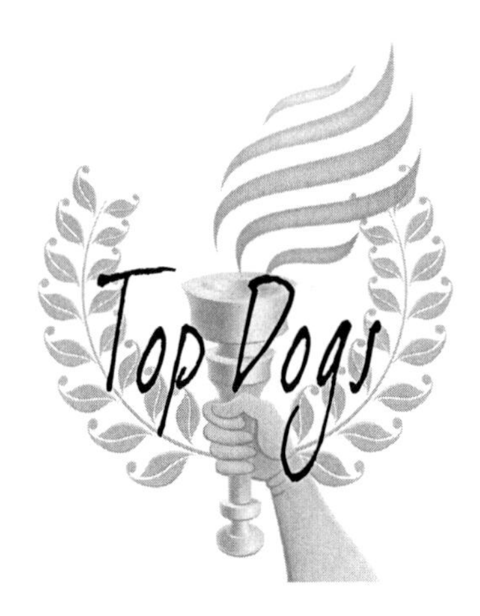

"Scott, you'll never guess what happened," Suzy said as I arrived at the rink. It was my first day back. "It's totally awesome."

Before I could fashion an answer, I heard Luddy's voice beckoning me.

"Scott!" I looked down the rink-side and saw him motioning me to his office.

As I walked past the bleachers, I felt slightly curious that Suzy would hear some awesome news before I did.

"So, how are you feeling?" Luddy asked as he closed the door behind me.

"A bit stiff," I said, "but it's still in there."

"What?" Luddy sounded concerned.

"Yeah," I continued. "They tried to unscrew it, but it wouldn't budge. So they snapped the ends off each side and now I'm fine."

Luddy shook his head. "So, have you started listening to music?"

"Yeah," I replied, "I have it with me. Do you have time to listen to it?"

Luddy took the tape from me and dropped it in the cassette player. Suddenly, parts of "The Sabre Dance," an upbeat Russian piece, filled the room. I watched Luddy closely as he listened. When his head started nodding while keeping time with the music, I knew I was home free.

"Good," he said. "By the way, the Delaware Symphony wants to compose your free-dance and record it live."

"What?" I couldn't believe what I was hearing.

"Yeah," he continued. "It's never been done. It's going to be great."

"What do you mean?"

"You know that Stephen Gunzenhauser's daughter is skating here," Luddy began, settling back in his chair.

"Yeah. Isn't he the conductor of the Delaware Symphony? We went to a party at his house."

"Good memory," Luddy said.

"Yeah, I like him. He's got a lot of good energy."

"He came up with this idea of the symphony recording a piece for one of my top skaters. You are the obvious pick."

Luddy's words floored me. Is that how he saw me? Is that how others saw me? I'd only been with him for four years. How did that happen?

"Regionals aren't that far away," he continued. "Since you and Suzy are a new team, we want next year to be special—to open the season with something new and fresh. This is the perfect showcase to get the program out there."

Luddy's affirmations, while encouraging, were also scary. Sure, Peter and Kitty Caruthers had retired, along with other top skaters on Luddy's team. Then it hit me for the first time. Peter told me that it would be my turn one day, but was this it?

"Scott? Scott!" Luddy said, awakening me from my daydream.

I shook my head.

"I'm sorry . . ." I hesitated. "It just hit me. Most of my peers have gone on—Lisa to school, Peter and Kitty to the Ice Capades, and, well, there aren't a whole lot left."

Luddy chuckled.

"I'm serious!" I felt slightly panicked. The peace that I felt when I was on the lake lingered somewhere in the back of my mind. *Should I have turned pro? Should I have* . . . I stopped speculating. It was my decision to find a new partner and start all over again. Luddy wasn't the one: it was me. And now I had dragged a relative novice into the limelight. Was this fair to her? I remembered how shaky I felt when Lisa and I came to Wilmington. Is that how Suzy felt?

"I have one question for you," Luddy leaned forward with a twinkle in his eye. "Have you accomplished everything you thought you should? Have you done all you expected?"

I breathed deeply, my doubts slipping away.

"No, sir, I haven't. I want to win Nationals and maybe even an Olympic medal. But how will that happen if we don't make the World team this year? You know how it is—out of sight, out of mind. We've got to go to the Worlds. That took Lisa and me two years."

"Suzy isn't Lisa," Luddy said quietly. "I've been watching her."

"Yeah—and?"

"She's intense. She wants it just as badly as you do. That's why you two will be a good team. She may have to pace herself a bit differently than she has in the past, but she'll come around with a little more experience."

"So, I suppose it's time to get back on the ice."

"You've got a lot of ground to cover," Luddy said as we stood up. I glanced at my watch.

"Time for your next lesson?"

Luddy chuckled as he walked to the door. "How many people get to do what they love to do 24/7?" he asked as he stepped over the threshold.

I retrieved the cassette, dropped it into my bag, and headed out the door. Stepping across the threshold, my mood greatly improved. I knew that I had made the right choice.

Luddy took the tape to Stephen the next day. By the time we met with him the following week, Jeffrey Budin, his arranger, had already scored the piece. We were about to begin a whole new artistic experience.

There's a surge of familiarity I feel when I walk through the doors of an ice rink, whether it's in my hometown or someplace more exotic like Tokyo or Sarejevo. The slightly musty smell shaved by the crisp, clean scent of freshly Zambonied ice heightens my sense of anticipation for what's next. But walking into Wilmington's Grand Opera House was different. The muffled, muted sense of raw artistry seemed to drip from every carpet fiber and the walls themselves. The low ceilings were totally opposite to our skating environment, yet the closed-in feeling wasn't restrictive. It was like being in a very precious music box, snuggled in and secure. I felt calm and relaxed, ready to try something new and different.

Although it was renovated in 1971, I still got a sense of the Grand Opera House's rich history. This was the home of the Delaware Symphony Orchestra.

Without saying a word, we made our way into the theatre and took our seats about six rows back, traditionally the best in the house for both visual and acoustical effect. Before we got too comfortable, Stephen came out to greet us.

"It's good to see you again," he said, warmth exuding from his voice.

"Thank you," I replied, still sensing the awe of our surroundings. I couldn't think of anything profound to say, so I stayed quiet.

"I'm glad you could make it," Stephen said as the orchestra members took their places on stage. After instructing us on how and when to make suggestions, Stephen took his place on stage with his musicians, who started playing.

"Unbelievable," I muttered as the richly textured sound surrounded me. Nothing electronic could come close to re-creating the dynamics of this live performance. As they continued playing, I closed my eyes so I could watch our rehearsed movement in my mind.

Suddenly, I lost the beat. I could visualize the movements; however, the music didn't match. Something was missing, but what?

"Drums!" I whispered to Jeffrey, who was sitting in the seat in front of us. "We need more drums here."

He silently nodded and made a notation on the sheet music in front of him.

I listened closely, comparing it to the music that was playing in my head.

"The pace is off a little here," I continued.

"Yeah, it needs to be faster," Suzy said, her eyes glistening with unshed tears. "This is awesome," she whispered.

I nodded, as much into the piece now as I was when I was making the changes for the cassette production. "Higher here," I whispered. "Let it build a bit faster because we do a lift here."

Jeffrey took every note with precision and understanding. Soon, his pristine sheet of music paper looked like chickens had danced across them. I don't know how long we worked together like that, but by the end of the process, we had a danceable routine—one that matched what we had been practicing for the last few weeks. This was the first of several meetings. When the music was complete, we left inspired and eager.

In my quiet time on the lake in Skaneateles, I felt destined to remain on the amateur circuit for another four years. Starting the season with a new partner and blending a previously untapped art form with skating confirmed that I was on the right track.

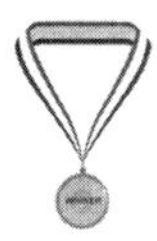

We planned to inaugurate the Delaware Symphony piece at the South Atlantic Regional Competition. Our practice sessions were spent not only in learning the routines but also in finding our rhythm and flow. I thought we had worked it all out, but I didn't take our nervous energy into account. Our compulsories at Regionals were shaky, especially when Suzy came toward me so hard at the end of our first dance that she almost knocked me down. But it didn't take long for her to find her stride. By the time we did our free dance, her energy was settled, so she was skating clean. Despite our rough start, we still managed to get enough points to win the competition.

A few weeks later we were skating at the Eastern Sectionals in Lake Placid, New York. We did well and qualified for the U. S. National Figure Skating Championships in Kansas City. Placing here would qualify us for the Worlds in Tokyo, Japan, in early March.

Suzy's confidence was so high that she was absolutely soaring. This was even better than she'd hoped. We were counting on Tokyo, but we had not figured on the unexpected.

Winters in the Midwest can be brutal, especially in Kansas City. When we arrived, I felt fine. Our practice sessions went well, even though I felt rather sluggish. No one else noticed, but I did. I dismissed it as jet lag and focused instead on preparing for the competition. By mid-week, I knew that I was in trouble. My energy was dropping steadily, and I didn't know if it was the flu or a bad cold. Whatever it was, I knew I was in for a bad time. To make matters worse, I couldn't medicate myself with over-the-counter drugs or anything. We were all drug-tested at the end of the competition. Even a cold remedy from the drugstore could show up on the tests and disqualify us, regardless of our standing.

After talking with Robbie and Luddy, I decided that practicing was more important than resting. I needed to get familiar with the rink, but I didn't realize how wiped out I was.

"Scott, we're here," Suzy said as we pulled up to the convention center.

"What?" I'd been dozing on the ride from the hotel.

"Can you skate?" Suzy asked.

"Yeah," I groaned as I stood up and stepped into the aisle. "It's just a cold."

She put her hand on my forehead, like my mother did when I was a kid. "You're burning up!"

"I'll be fine," I choked out with a cough stuck in my throat. Suzy stepped off the bus. Looking back at me, she almost ran into a signpost.

"Suzy, I've skated when I felt a lot worse than I do now," I groused. I was having trouble keeping my patience in check. "We don't always get to do this when we're a hundred percent. You focus on getting ready, and I'll do the same." As I paused for a moment, a light-headed wave curled over my head. I took a deep breath and stepped alongside her. "I'll do the same after I take a bit of a rest in the locker room. Have Robbie come get me five minutes before our practice program starts."

Before Suzy could say anything else, I headed toward the men's locker room, put on my practice clothes and skates, and laid down on the bench. I was vaguely aware of activity going on around me as competitors came and left. "That should be me," I argued with my body. "Why won't you move?" But my body wasn't listening. Moments later, I drifted off.

"Scott?" a male voice broke into my haze. "Scott?" This time he seemed a bit louder. It was Robbie.

"What?" I was confused. I didn't know where I was.

"You're going to be up soon," he said as he helped me up. "Let's get you on the ice."

"Thanks," I said, taking a deep breath. "I'll be all right."

When I joined Suzy in the arena, she looked flushed and psyched. She'd been warming up by herself. The moment she saw me, her whole countenance changed.

"Suzy," I kept my voice even and strong. "Focus! I'll do my part. Just make sure you do yours."

During the time that followed, I drew on every bit of energy I could muster and then offered a quick prayer asking for even more. The music began, and my adrenaline started pumping.

Our run-through for our four minute program went well, much to Suzy's surprise. Then *boom*, I was off the ice. I was done. I forfeited some of our practice time, but Suzy could use it if she wanted. I needed to rest because I just couldn't muster up any more energy.

As soon as we returned to the hotel, I ate a quick dinner and then went to bed. Despite my bravado in front of Suzy, I was beginning to wonder if I would make it through the rest of the week. I didn't sleep well, so when my roommate Todd came in, I knew it was time to try something more drastic. I took my bedding into the bathroom and made a place to sleep on the floor. Then, I turned on the shower to generate steam, hoping this would improve my breathing, and fell asleep.

About four a.m., someone pounding on our door awakened me. The steam fog was so thick that I couldn't see anything clearly. Two hotel security guards emerged from the mist with Todd trailing behind them. No one looked happy. Unfortunately, my makeshift steam room had set off a smoke alarm; but on the plus side, I felt better.

The next day, our competition began. After we completed our final dance, our scores lit up across the rink. We placed well. I was returning to the locker room when one of the judges stopped me.

"It really looks good, Scott," he said. "You've worked hard, and it shows."

"Thank you," I said.

"You've got a real dynamo there," he continued, chatting about Suzy's enthusiasm and skill.

"It was a good move," I replied. Moments later, he was heading back to the judge's room.

Suzy and I lost the U. S. silver medal to Renee Roca and Donald Adair by one-tenth of a point. Even though we didn't have any mistakes during the competition, we walked away with a bronze, thanks to one judge. Doing this well with less than six months together positioned us to do even better next year.

Our bronze medal ensured us a place on the World team going to Tokyo. We were on our way. I did it: I accomplished one of my goals with a new partner—getting right back on the World team without missing a year. Perseverance had paid off.

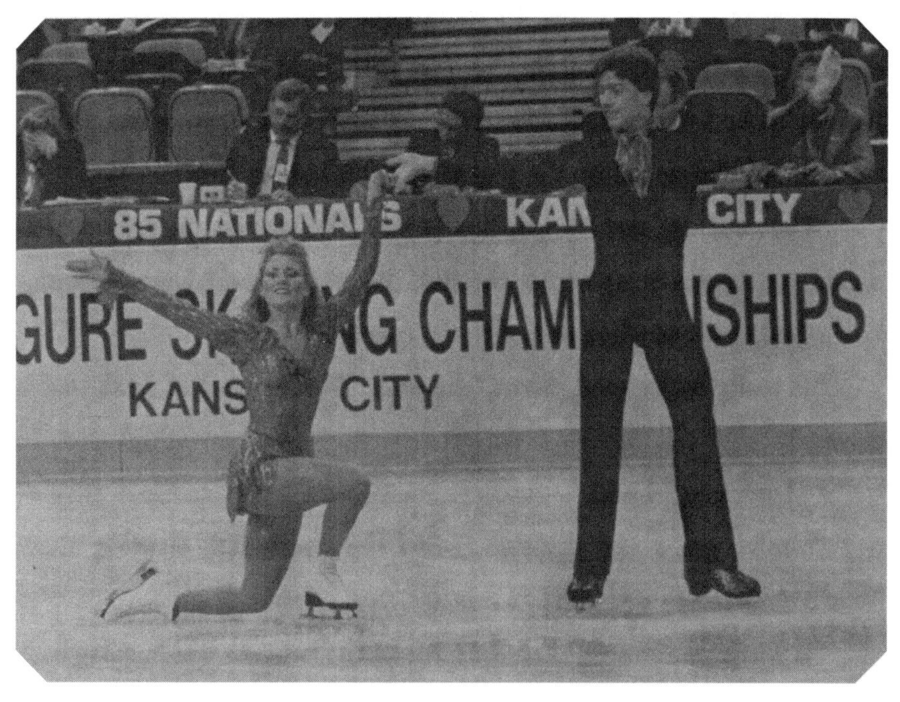

Reveling in the applause as Suzy and I compete at our first Nationals in 1985.

Chapter 22

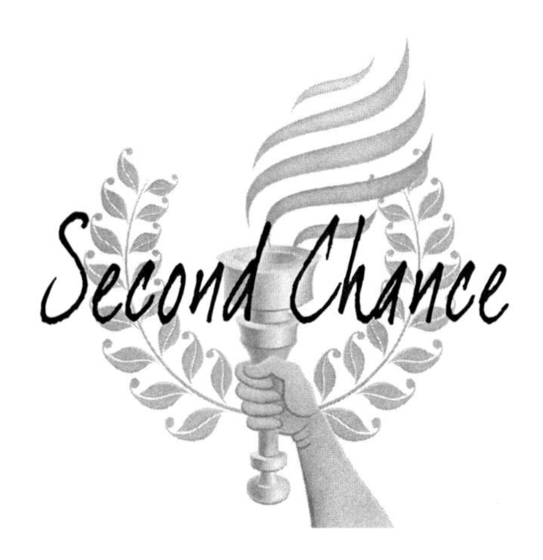

Second Chance

With our good showing at Nationals, Suzy and I were well on our way. She fully adjusted to the crazy training schedule at the Skating Club of Wilmington. As one of the top training centers in the country because of Luddy, the rink was filled for most of the sessions with competitive skaters. We still needed more ice time, so I immediately thought of Havertown.

Our typical day started at 9:30 a.m. with a forty-five minute drive to Havertown. After two hours in the almost-empty rink, we returned to Wilmington for ninety minutes on the ice at our home club. During that time, we spent about half an hour with Luddy. Afterwards, we participated in group dance lessons for an hour, followed by drama classes and weight-lifting—anything to help improve our skills. At 5 p.m., we finished our daytime routine. I went home, fixed dinner, napped for two hours, and returned to the rink by 10:45, ready for the next round. We kept this schedule for two years.

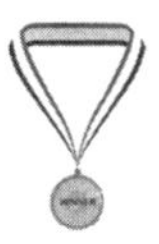

We were at the top of our game when we went to Worlds in Tokyo in March, 1985. We were in tenth place for the first part of the competition—not where I wanted to be, but considering it was our first year, it wasn't too shabby. When it was time for our free dance, however, everything changed. It was one of those chance blips that we had hoped to avoid: we stumbled slightly. Yet, the result was devastation, because we dropped to twelfth place. To me, that was like getting a C-minus or D on a school report card.

Sitting in the kiss-and-cry area while watching our tenth place position slip away, it was obvious to those around us that we weren't happy. Suzy was close to tears because she was so mad. We stood to return to the changing areas.

"Hey, guys," Luddy said. "What's your problem here?"

Neither of us uttered a word, so Luddy walked alongside us.

"It's too bad you had the mishap in the last ten seconds of your free dance. But don't worry about it, and don't dwell on it. You've only been together for less than a year. Suzy, how many competitors are at Worlds in less than a year?"

Suzy's frustration began to seep away.

"And Scott, you know better. You've always been a good sport and risen above the setbacks. Forget about this, and just do better next time."

Luddy's positive words pulled us back on track quickly and reminded us to focus forward rather than to dwell on one mistake. By the time we reached the changing rooms, we both felt better and encouraged. Suzy and I returned to our off-season schedule in Wilmington, which wasn't quite as rigorous as the regular training. We'd been at it about a month when we got our second chance.

"Scott, Suzy, come here!" Luddy's voice boomed across the rink.

We stopped abruptly, saw him standing on the walkway next to the bleachers, and skated toward him.

"Great news," Luddy said as we approached the boards. "You need to pack your bags."

"Where are we going?" Suzy asked.

"Morzine," he said, looking quite content.

"France?" Momentarily speechless, I noted my heart pounding, and panic threatened to override logic. It couldn't be possible, could it? "What happened?"

"One of the American teams dropped out."

"But that's only ten days away!" Suzy shrieked.

"Yep," Luddy said. "Bring your free dance music in tonight, and we'll start your run-throughs. See you at 11."

Suzy and I stood at the rail, stunned as Luddy turned and started to walk away.

"Do you want to do this?" he asked.

"Of course we do," both Suzy and I replied, without even consulting each other.

He continued his walk to his office. "Now get back to work."

The next ten days were a whirlwind. Trying to make up for lost time, we practiced with greater intensity than ever before. It was hard enough just getting through the programs again because we had been away from them for so long. We didn't have the luxury of gradually preparing for the event. We pushed so hard that I felt nauseous during some of the practices, but today I don't regret one moment of it. I was determined to do better at Morzine to redeem myself.

Morzine was unbelievably gorgeous. We stayed at the bottom of a mountain in a ski resort at a first-class French chalet. It quickly ranked high on my list of favorite places to visit.

Much to everyone's surprise, including ours, we came in first. That competition was a turning point for us, putting us higher than teams who placed seventh and eighth at Worlds. I was on top of the world for the next twenty-four hours.

On the day after the competition, we were supposed to skate in a closing exhibition. Suzy and I skated our winning program, but we made a slight mistake during the routine. It wasn't *that* noticeable, but to the experienced eye of an official with the International Skating Union, it was glaring. He stopped me after the show.

"Scott, wait a minute," he said as I was walking down the hall to the locker room. I turned and waited for him to speak.

"You've got what it takes," he said. "You two have to keep working at it. I can see you at the top someday, but you can't go out there and make errors—not even a little mistake."

I felt like he'd hit me with a sledge hammer. I must have had a rather dumbfounded expression on my face because he continued.

"If you want to be a champion, you cannot make mistakes at any time. Do you understand?"

I was floored, but he was right. I understood something then that I had been taking for granted.

"Yes, sir," I said quietly. "I . . . Thank you." His words turned a light bulb on in my mind.

Champions are always on their game because they're always focused on perfection. For them, an exhibition is just as important as a competition. A lack of focus and the added pressure of performing open the door for potential mistakes. To avoid them, we needed to be as intense in our training as we were in competition. We thought we were doing that already, but this experience just proved to us that there was more we could do.

His words became my mental mantra. The heady win and the judge's advice stoked our excitement. We encouraged each other, committing to perform from start to finish without any mistakes. This mantra became our common language. We would spot our trouble areas in a routine, talk it through, and correct it. We verbally reinforced both my job and hers.

"I'm going to remember to deepen my edge a little more while you keep yours the same so we don't run into each other," I would tell her before we started one of our moves. And that's how she knew I was correcting myself even more than I was correcting her. This heightened communication helped to increase our understanding and upped the ante.

When we couldn't be on the ice, we would go upstairs to the ballet room and work in front of the mirrors to double-check our timing and body lines. More time spent on connecting our movements zoned and sharpened our edge. Suzy and I were on the same page. As a team, we were willing to do what it took to win.

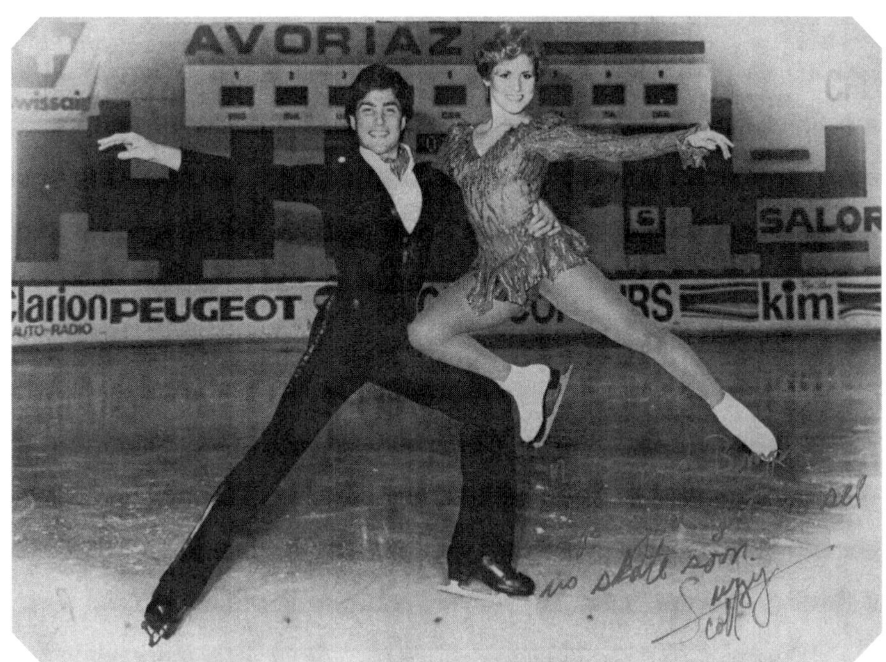

Suzy and I in Morzine, France, where we competed and redeemed our standing.

Chapter 23

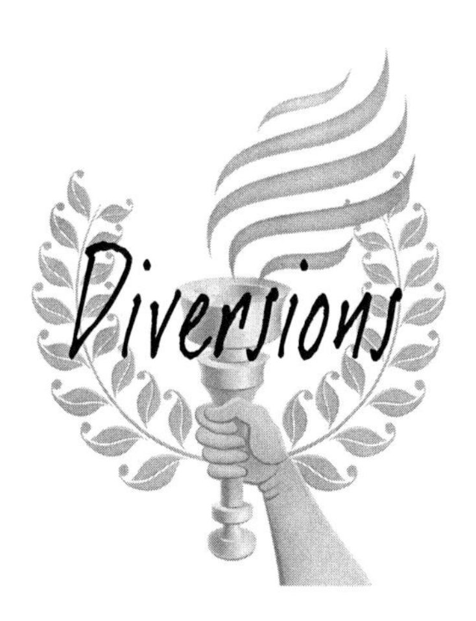

Life at 1430 Foulk Road was going well, too. I was taking a photography class at Philadelphia's Institute of the Arts. I enjoyed photography because it flexed my different creative muscles. One day I was driving through one of the Wilmington suburbs and passed this huge house. At the curbside, there was a big pile of stuff beside some garbage bins. On top was a ten-foot countertop, complete with a stainless-steel sink. It would be the perfect centerpiece for the darkroom I was planning to build. I immediately pulled over and got out of my car.

I looked the countertop over, and it seemed to be in pretty good condition. So, I walked up to the front porch and rang the bell. A well-dressed, middle-aged woman opened the door.

"Uh, my name's Scott Gregory, and I just saw the stainless-steel countertop at the end of your driveway. Are you throwing that away?"

"Yes," she replied.

"Would you mind if I come back in a couple hours and picked it up?"

"I don't see why not. Why don't you move it to the other side of the driveway to separate it from the rest of the trash?"

"I will. Thank you," I said as I turned away and jogged back to my newfound treasure.

It was heavier than I expected, but I did manage to drag it to the other side. Then I returned home to see if Todd was around. Next, we borrowed a truck from another friend and came back, hoping the sink would still be there.

I held my breath as we turned the corner, almost afraid that someone else had claimed my treasure, but it was still there! We loaded the sink on the truck and drove back to the house, where Todd and I unloaded the monster. We carried it downstairs and put it in the corner, across from the slideboard, a huge sheet of plywood covered with a wide strip of linoleum. It was designed for off-ice training and conditioning and also helped with stroking motions. Peter and I built one similar to five-time gold medalist Eric Heiden's design.

While we had the truck, we drove to the lumber yard and purchased everything else I needed. Before the weekend was over, I had created a first-class darkroom. Well, maybe it wasn't first class, but it suited me perfectly. I used a garden hose for water and let the sink drain into a bucket, but that didn't matter to me. It was my darkroom—my escape from the daily pressures of skating.

The U. S. Olympic Committee regularly helped its athletes find work. These contract jobs often helped us support some of the expenses associated with our sport. One of the work assignments I received was for a businessman in Philadelphia. He wanted me to photograph a specific group of buildings around Independence Hall so he could frame them for his office building.

Photography became my fantasy world, a place to visit for a glimpse of a larger world beyond the ice. I even considered becoming a professional photographer once I retired from the amateur arena. As much as I enjoyed photography, however, it wasn't my passion. The call of the ice was just too strong for me.

Since the Wilmington teams did so well in the 1984 Olympics, Luddy was looking for better ice times for his kids: us. That came in 1986, when the University of Delaware offered to build a second training rink for Luddy. In the meantime, we trained in the old rink while the new one was being built. Our training day started with a 6 a.m. wake-up call. Now, we no longer had to deal with driving to Havertown for ice time, skating in overcrowded conditions, and working around social skaters' schedules.

Our on-ice training now started around 7:30 a.m., and we remained at the rink until 3 p.m., when our off-ice routine began. Since I knew some of the doctors at A. I. duPont Hospital for Children, Suzy and I were allowed to do our weight-training in the hospital's rehab room for free. When we discovered that the university was offering drama classes, we jumped at the chance to attend because it would give us one more tool for our arsenal. We finished up around 5 p.m.

One of the best aspects about this new schedule revolved around our evenings. For the first time in seven years, my evenings were open, so we had time to relax and rest. One evening I was sitting in the living room at home watching CNN.

"Scott! What are you doing?"

Todd's voice drew me from the images of President Ronald Reagan's latest take on the Cold War.

"I'm watching the news."

"You're not ready?" Todd sounded petulant, like I had forgotten something important.

"Ready for what?"

"We're picking up the girls and some other skaters to go to Oscar's."

"What are you talking about?"

"Suzy didn't tell you?"

"Tell me what?"

"One of the kids in the drama class told her about this great place to get all-you-can-eat tacos for ninety-nine cents. It's in downtown Wilmington."

I thought hard but didn't remember a thing. Still, ninety-nine cent tacos sounded affordable. "Give me five minutes," I said as I turned off the television and raced upstairs to change clothes. A half-hour later, our cars were filled with passengers, and we were headed for what appeared to be a deserted area in downtown Wilmington. My enthusiasm for the restaurant was quickly waning.

"Where is this place supposed to be?" I asked.

"Market Street," Suzy replied.

"This place doesn't look too—"

"Come on, Scott," Suzy interrupted. "I'm hungry!"

As I got out of the car, I glanced at Todd. He was as uncertain as I was about the lack of light and bodies. But the girls were fearless, so we followed them, casually looking over our shoulders to make sure no one was scoping us out.

As we walked along the brick sidewalk, dusk was rapidly fading into darkness. The lack of lighting added an almost spooky feeling to our lone walk.

"Todd, are you sure this place is on Market Street?" I whispered as I quick-stepped to catch up with him.

"Creepy, isn't it?"

"Here it is!" Kristan, another roommate, called out before I could respond.

The windows were dark, so we couldn't see inside.

"Are they open?" I wasn't sure about this, but I was hungry too. "It looks like an old bank."

I opened the door, and the eight of us crossed the threshold. It was a complete contrast to the dark, deserted streets outside. Huge paintings lined the walls, giving it a larger-than-life effect. Warm laughter, underscored by the soft buzz of fluorescent lights, added to the welcoming atmosphere. A bar to the left offered just about everything we couldn't have since we were in training. Seating on both the main floor and the balcony promised excellent opportunities for people-watching while diners enjoyed their meals. The Wednesday night taco special seemed to draw a younger crowd, and the price was right.

"How many?" asked a tall, middle-aged woman with dark hair greeting us at the door.

"Eight," I replied. "Could we sit in the balcony?"

Moments later, we were seated above the crowd. They pushed two tables together to accommodate our group. There was no need to look at the menu because we knew what we wanted.

"I'm Connie. I'll be your waitress tonight. What would you like to order?"

"Tacos!" we said in unison. From that night on, Oscar's became our favorite Wednesday-night hangout. No one knew who we were or what we did, which was refreshing. We always sat in the balcony. The next day, we were back at the rink and ready to go.

Chapter 24

Since our training schedule was more efficient, it gave us additional creative time to build and develop our programs. Soon it was time for Nationals in Uniondale, New York, during a cold February in 1986. Without the previous year's champions competing, first place was well within our reach, especially since our first compulsory dance went so well. Our second compulsory dance was another story.

Suzy and I were the last team to skate. After so many teams had skated the same pattern, the ice had become very rutty. Although I was focused on the dance, I failed to compensate for the depth of the grooves in the ice. I slightly stumbled, which I immediately corrected. Even though I didn't fall, the bobble caught the judges' eyes. That slip was enough to overshadow the rest of the competition for us and open the door for the other team to move ahead of us into first place.

I need to get it together. I've got to get my head in the game for the rest of the competition. Even though my head-talk improved my performance attitude and we skated clean for the remaining events, we still ended up in second place. It was a split score with the judges, and some people say that we should have won. One simple mistake, however, was enough to take us down a notch. It wasn't a matter of anyone's fault; we just failed to adapt our program to the deeper grooves in the ice, which threw us off.

To fuel my frustration, Todd and his partner, Gillian, won in the pairs division. He was on top of the world, but I was so miserable that I couldn't be the friend to him that I should have been. Instead of rejoicing with him, I grudgingly congratulated my best friend and then went off to sulk. I should have been on top like Todd, sharing and celebrating the championship together.

The next major event was Worlds in Geneva. I was determined to train past the mistake by perfecting our rhythm and timing. We decided that we were going to do much better than Nationals, and we did. No bobbles plagued us that time. We came in fifth, placing ahead of the team who beat us at Nationals, so we jumped up seven spots from last year's placement.

It didn't take long to wrap my mind around placing fifth at Worlds, my highest ranking so far. We were on a roll, but it wasn't until a few days later when we took a well-earned and much-needed ski vacation in a small town called Arolla in Switzerland that I realized I was becoming one of the best ice dancers in the world. It was a cool feeling.

My parents had planned the ski trip, and Suzy, Gillian, and her parents came along. We stayed in a mountain chalet that had a gorgeous view of the ragged, towering peaks of the Pennine Alps.

To reach the top of the slopes, we had to drive up a long, narrow road winding up the hill through tunnels in the sides of the mountain and steep inclines without guardrails. As passengers, we got the chance to enjoy a panorama that was incredible beyond all imagination. The driver, however, wasn't so fortunate. Had he taken his eyes off the road, we would have been a goner.

Once at the top, the view was awesome. The mountains were huge, and the ski trails were open slopes all the way down. When I pointed to some helicopters dropping explosives in the snow on the opposite mountain for avalanche control, our group stopped. We were close enough to see the pilots and hear the explosives' muffled rumble in the valley below. I found the whole process fascinating. Nevertheless, in spite of man's intervention, the mountain's majesty remained overwhelming and breath-taking.

Being able to relax and enjoy the country was a treat. Usually my visits to other nations were limited to skating, eating, sleeping, and then skating some more. Then, *boom*! I was back home. But this was different. Being in those mountains helped keep everything in perspective by making me appreciate the fact that I could travel all over the world and enjoy my efforts of hard, dedicated work at the same time.

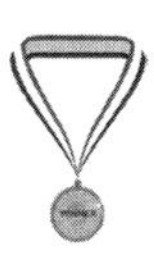

Satisfied and refreshed, we returned to Wilmington, looking forward to the more relaxed exhibition schedule.

Part of that schedule included an invitation to participate in the first Goodwill Games in Moscow. Created as a way to ease tensions during the Cold War through friendly sports competition between nations, the 1986 Games featured more than 3,000 world-class athletes from 79 countries, competing in 182 gold-medal events in 18 sports. Figure skating was one of the events featured on the schedule.

Of course, not every trip to compete runs smoothly. Anything can happen, and it did during a short layover in Düesseldorf, Germany, en route to our final destination in Moscow.

Todd sat at a window seat, watching the luggage being loaded. I was next to him, casually leafing through the airline magazine. I had started reading an article on the first leg that I wanted to finish.

"I wonder what they're doing," Todd said rather nonchalantly.

"Who?"

"Those guards around the luggage."

I leaned over him to look out the window. The luggage carrier was stopped, and some Russian guards were pulling one of the bags off the trolley and onto the ground. As officers of the Russian embassy, part of their task was ensuring the security of flights heading into their country.

"Hey! That looks like one of my bags," I said.

"How can you tell?" Todd asked. "All I see are three Russian guards with guns pointing at it."

"Attention!"

We looked up and saw a Russian military officer with a rifle over his shoulder. His heavily-accented question gained our full attention.

"Whose bag?" he demanded, pointing out the window.

I looked around and tentatively raised my hand.

"Come with me!"

I looked at Todd, gulped, and stood to follow the officer. As I walked down the aisle, my imagination went into overdrive. Scenes of being dragged off to jail despite my pleas to call the American embassy played out a hundred different ways. Walking down the steps onto the tarmac, I felt my heart starting to beat louder. As we closed in on the errant bag, I was hoping that they were mistaken. My hopes were dashed when I saw it because I knew for sure that it was mine. Then I heard it. A low buzzing noise was emanating from its depths.

"Open bag," my captor demanded. Kneeling slowly, I zipped open the soft-sided luggage.

One of the soldiers leaned over and started poking my clothing with his rifle when he uncovered the source of the strange noise. At some point during the trip, my luggage must have jostled, turning on my battery-operated razor.

"Razor," I muttered with a sickly smile as I reached over and turned it off. "Sorry."

My guard took it from my hands, examined it thoroughly, and then tossed it back into my bag. After I closed the case, luggage handlers came back out and started loading the plane.

"Come with me," the guard replied as he escorted me back to the aircraft.

"Thanks," I replied, catching a glimpse of one of the younger guards. He was obviously working hard to suppress a chuckle as they turned to march back to the terminal. As I returned to my seat, my teammates applauded my performance. They were probably thinking, *Scott has done it again!*

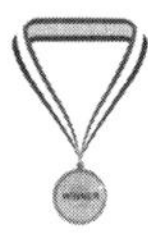

The first thing I noticed when we got off the plane in Moscow was that everything was gray and drab. Todd and I both felt like we were in a Cold War movie because soldiers with machine guns were everywhere. The hotel was depressing. Feeling uncomfortable and out of place, we even wondered if our room was bugged.

The food we ate in the buffet-style hotel restaurant was—well, let's say, interesting. I think the chef must have been writing a book entitled *101 Russian Ways to Cook Goulash*, and we got to taste ninety-nine of them. We didn't have to worry about gaining weight that trip.

Suzy's Russian heritage, on the other hand, helped her feel right at home. Her favorite part was our chance to skate with Andrei Bukin and his partner, Natalia Bestemianova. They were the world champions, and we were the up-and-coming young team. One of the dances we skated to was "The Killian," during which we switched partners while skating side by side. I teamed up with Natalia, and Suzy went with Andrei. Fortunately, they spoke English, so we could communicate. Our international dance was performed to demonstrate the concept that when the world gets together and works together, we can produce beautiful things. For me, it was quite a paradigm shift. All I wanted to do was beat the Russians because they were so good.

The next day, while practicing a sequence in our show number, Suzy and I had an accident. During this dance, I would do a somersault on the ice. As I rolled over, Suzy would straddle over me and glide away in the opposite direction. This time, however, we mistimed our movement. As I rolled out of the somersault, my momentum stopped abruptly when my heel caught her buttocks, cutting in a good inch. Blood, lots of it, gushed everywhere, and she screamed.

"Oh, my God," I cried. "Suzy! You're—" I couldn't finish my sentence. My partner crumbled on the ice, tears rolling down her cheeks. She couldn't talk because she could hardly breathe.

Unable to think of any way to stop the endless stream of blood pooling around her, I cradled her head in my lap as I looked up and around in disbelief for help.

Before she could say anything, all the other skaters gathered around her. A tall, blond guy pulled off his sweater and thrust it into my hands.

"Wrap this around to stop the bleeding," he said, his Russian accent barely noticeable.

"Here," another skater said as she knelt down and gently placed her sweater underneath Suzy's head. More sweaters and towels were put in place, slowing the free flow of blood tinting the ice.

Suzy grabbed my hand but still couldn't say anything, and I looked around helplessly. Thankfully, our team doctor, Howard Silby, was rushing across the ice toward us, carrying towels.

"She, I—"

"I saw," he said, cutting off additional any comments. He pressed towels against her backside to slow down the flow of blood and helped carry her onto the side benches. Suzy wouldn't let go of my hand; her grip was like a vise.

The bumpy ambulance ride to the clinic seemed to take hours. When they took her into the dark, gray cinderblock building, I expected to see brightly-lit, ultra-sanitary facilities that we're used to in the States. But it was the opposite, seeming almost primitive and unsanitary. Much to my surprise, the ambulance driver took Suzy into a treatment room, washed his hands, and acted like he was going to stitch up her wound.

"You're the doctor?" I exclaimed, feeling even more uneasy than before.

"Scott, wait outside," Dr. Silby said, firmly.

"But—" The look on his face and the tone of his voice commanded obedience. "I'll be right outside," I said to Suzy, who was clammy and pale. She nodded her head. "Dr. Silby is here. He'll take care of you." She nodded again. I felt her hand release mine as I backed out of the room.

I was seated alone in that dingy, cold waiting room, where I started beating myself up for what happened. Had I mistimed my movements, or had she? What difference did it make, though? She was hurt anyway. Was she injured too badly to skate in the exhibition that night?

As I was debating the need to skate, Dr. Silby joined me in the waiting room.

"She's going to be sore, but she'll be fine," he said. "We managed to get the bleeding stopped and her wound stitched. She's determined to skate tonight."

"Really?" I said, surprised by Suzy's determination. I stood up. "She's able to skate?"

"She's going to be fine," Dr. Silby finished. "She might be in pain, and if it opens up a little, we'll have to restitch it."

"Yeah, but she . . . are you sure?"

"Scott, I'm skating," Suzy said as she wobbled into the waiting room. "I'll be fine, but you're a mess!" She grabbed my arm and leaned heavily on me as we returned to the ambulance for the long journey back. I couldn't argue with her.

Our return trip to the hotel was much faster than our ride out. After a few hours' rest, Suzy said she felt strong enough to skate. So that night we were back in our places on time and ready to go. Suzy was stiff and in pain as we started our number, but she continued, resolute and focused on finishing. All I could do was stand by and remain doubly focused, while making sure nothing else happened to her.

Our three minute exhibition number to Barbra Streisand's hit "Somewhere" seemed to be over in thirty seconds. Suzy was a real trouper and champion, and it showed in her performance. The Russian audience stood, which was a rare and unexpected response. I couldn't have been prouder of her. We skated with vigor to center ice to take our bows, and then skated off to the exit door and into the locker room, where Dr. Silby redressed her wound.

The next day, we left Russia. Our trip back to the States was uneventful, especially since I took the batteries out of my razor. Interacting with our Russian counterparts and sharing their concern when Suzy was laying on the ice spoke volumes about our common experience. We came as tentative strangers and left as friends. For me, as an American, it was an honor to perform in Russia, spending time with fellow American skaters and building a bond. What rich memories! Now I was ready for the next big hurdle, a chance to win the U. S. Championships.

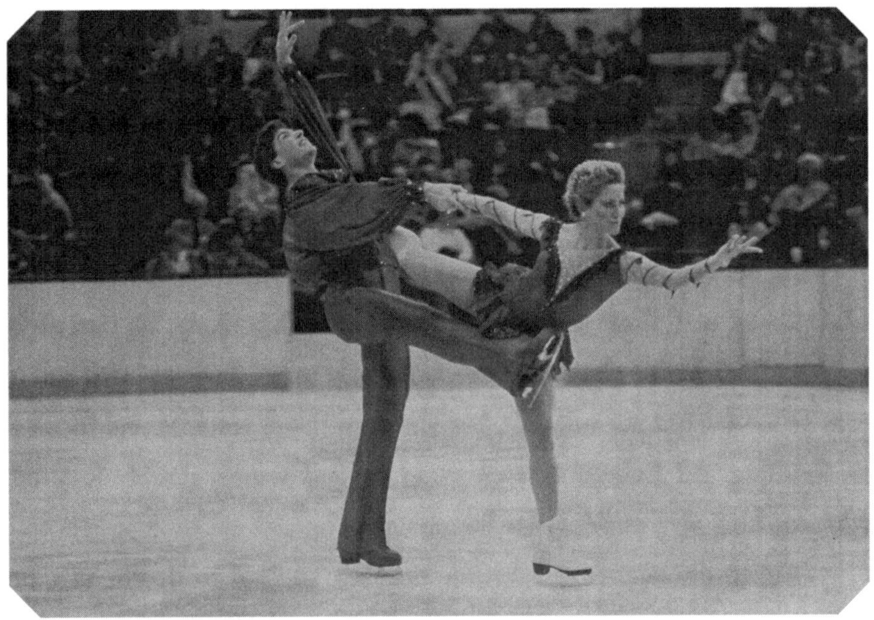

Suzy and I performing a maneuver we used in Moscow.

Chapter 25

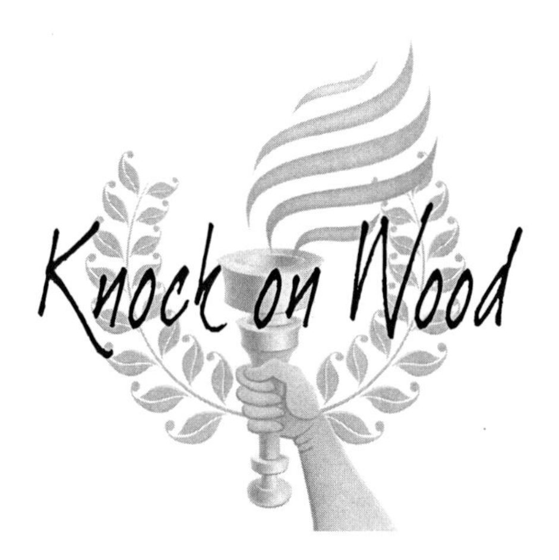

Knock on Wood

With the Goodwill Games behind us, we focused on preparing for the 1987 competition season. Finding the right music was always a difficult task. We wanted something unique and original that would engage both the audience and the judges. Suzy and I quickly agreed on the first two pieces for our free dance, with the song "Waiting for the Robert E. Lee" as our first choice. It was upbeat and segued well into the blues number that we found. But the choice of our closing number had us stumped. We wanted a great, powerful ending that would engage the audience. Finally we stumbled across a flute and guitar arrangement of "Dueling Banjos." It had the perfect blend of the unique and original, and clearly was the best conclusion to the Dixieland band theme we were building.

This free dance was more complex, required higher energy, and featured more intricate and difficult footwork than we had skated in previous competitions. The audience had to love it. Their approval and participation could well be a tie-breaker at Nationals.

With a chance to win so close, Suzy and I knew that we had to work smarter than ever before. We relied heavily on our choreographers, Diane Agle and Jill Cosgrove, to create the dance and our coaches, Luddy and Robby, to tweak our presentation. But this time, something was different; we felt as if a breakthrough was guaranteed.

A week before Nationals, all I wanted to do was get there. But then we kept practicing, fine-tuning, and finding the sweet spot of better. We didn't realize how sweet it was, until one of our last free dance run-throughs.

Skaters dotted our home rink, working on their own routines. While we were running through our program, the music for "Dueling Banjos" started. Out of respect, our fellow skaters moved off to the side. Pushing my focus back to our routine, I let myself fly with the tune. Sixty seconds later, it was over. Suzy looked up at me and then around.

"Oh!" she exclaimed. All of our friends were cheering and clapping.

"Wow, that was great," I said.

Suzy and I started our cool-down lap amid shouts of encouragement and pats on the back.

I heard Todd's voice first. "Great job!"

"Good free dance," Gillian's excitement was infectious, even though it didn't take too much to raise our excitement meter.

"What can be better than this?" Suzy whispered.

"Making it better," I replied, breathing heavily with my hands on my knees.

The next morning, we were on our way to Tacoma, Washington. It was a smooth flight with friendly stews and plenty of bantering among the Delaware contingency. Then I heard it: "ding ding," the two-bell signal to let us know we were descending. I looked out the window as the jet was angling down beneath the rainy clouds toward the Tacoma-Seattle Airport. As I looked toward the horizon, there it was—the Seattle skyline with the Space Needle and Mt. Rainier in the distance. Despite this gloomy weather that reminded me of Moscow, I was excited, for I had colossal expectations.

We quickly fell into the routine of practicing and familiarizing ourselves with the rink. Three days later, the competition began. We sailed through the compulsories and quickly established ourselves as the team to beat. I couldn't wait for Saturday night. I was anxious, excitedly anticipating our turn to take the ice. There is always the risk of becoming complacent when you're out front early in the game. One might think that because you are in first place heading into the last event, you could ease up and relax. But thinking that way would be the kiss of death.

Think positive, Scott. Stay focused. That mantra played and replayed itself through my mind's ear all week. If I lost my focus or intensity, I might have found myself totally off course, but I refused to stray. Everything was working as the week crawled toward the final events on Saturday. Containing my anticipation proved monumental as seconds ticked away in slow motion through the morning, past the afternoon, and well into the evening.

Finally, Suzy and I were on the ice, ready to skate after our six-minute warm-up. Before they called our names to be the next team, just like always, I needed to see where Mom and Dad were sitting in the packed house of twenty-three thousand. Dad promised to wear a uniquely designed "good luck sweater" I received at an international competition in Japan earlier that year. It was yellow with a "number one," a horseshoe, and an ace of diamonds playing card on it. I'm normally not superstitious, but I believed seeing Dad in that sweater would cinch it—I just knew it. The gold medal hinged on this one final performance, and I wanted all the odds in my favor.

I looked up in the stands, where every color under the rainbow glistened beneath the hot television lights. *How could I find a bright yellow sweater in this sea of hues?* My heart started pounding, and panic threatened to overwhelm me. *What if I couldn't see them? What if . . .* Suddenly, I saw this bright yellow sweater and arms waving. It was my dad standing there, with a big smile on his face. A barely perceptible light surrounded him. I looked closer, and it seemed like it was coming from above. Was this a sign? I looked at Suzy, who was pacing around, preparing for our free dance. I looked back at my dad, and the light was still around him. No one else may have seen it, but I did. I exhaled, realizing for the first time that I'd been holding my breath.

The announcer called our name, so it was time for us to turn it on. We got in position and waited for the signal to begin our program. I stood with my chest out, head up, and hands on my hips. Suzy knelt, with her face forward in front and head angled down. The music started, and we jumped into the routine that we had practiced for more than a hundred hours. Before I realized it, the familiar twang of "Dueling Banjos" started playing. With only a minute left in our performance, I could feel the crowd! They were into it as much as we were. Usually at this point I would feel fatigued, but the energy of the crowd was like rocket fuel igniting my legs. We hit our last lift, I set Suzy down, and we took our ending position.

The crowd's roar echoed around the arena, freezing the moment like the final goal in an upset win at the Super Bowl and the winning pitch in the World Series all rolled into one. We had connected with the audience. People had jumped to their feet, applauding. The moment imprinted itself on my mind and my heart. It was all I had hoped and dreamed for—and more.

This cheering crowd was totally over the edge. My emotions were mixed: I was elated, overwhelmed, and humbled by it all. I took Suzy's hand, and we skated back to the kiss-and-cry area, where we sat and waited for our scores. As each number was displayed, our first-place position was confirmed. A sports announcer thrust a microphone in front of us just as the last number appeared on the scoreboard.

Looking at each other, Suzy and I got lost in the moment. Excitement exploded! We jumped off the bench and started hugging each other and anyone else who was within arm's reach. The jubilant crowd cheered with us as Robbie and Luddy patted us on the back and joined our group hug. The weight was lifted. We won! We had really done it!

"That was some program," the announcer said, shoving his microphone closer.

"We hoped it would be," I replied.

As we answered his questions, I realized that I had done it. After ten years of working at this level, I had finally climbed to the top. I was the national champion, but I couldn't have done it without Judy, Lisa, or Suzy. I was grateful for each partner, my parents, and my coaches—for all of them at this one, precious, moving moment. I looked over the tops of the heads of my peers to see Todd standing in the distance, grinning from ear to ear. He knew what I was feeling, and he was genuinely happy for me. It was my time.

An announcement for the top-three winners to assemble for the presentation of medals interrupted the interview. Suzy and I held hands as we skated to the podium, where they called our names and presented us to the audience. It was surreal, almost like a dream, but I knew it was real. As one of the top officials placed the medal around my neck, flashes of the last ten years danced before my mind's eye. Then it was over and time to get to the business of the rest of the evening—celebrating our victory!

Luddy pulled me aside before we headed to the locker room.

"I've coached a lot of people to this place," Luddy said, "but this championship was one of the hardest earned."

"I was beginning to wonder if I would ever make it," I replied.

"It was well earned and well deserved," he said patting me on the back again. "I was always proud of you because you hung in there, and now you've got the prize." Luddy's words were more than an encouragement; they were the icing on the cake.

After we changed clothes, my parents met us outside the locker rooms. We began our celebration by making the rounds of room parties at the hotel, then started making phone calls to everyone we could think of. Aroung two a.m., my folks called it a night. But Suzy and I had too much adrenaline flowing. We were up all night celebrating, enjoying our ride on cloud nine. It seemed like everybody was celebrating with us.

At 2:00 on Sunday afternoon we were back on the ice for the traditional exhibition.

Even though we had been celebrating through the night, reality didn't sink in until I heard the announcer call us onto the ice: "And now, the 1987 National Ice-Dancing Champions, Suzanne Semanick and Scott Gregory."

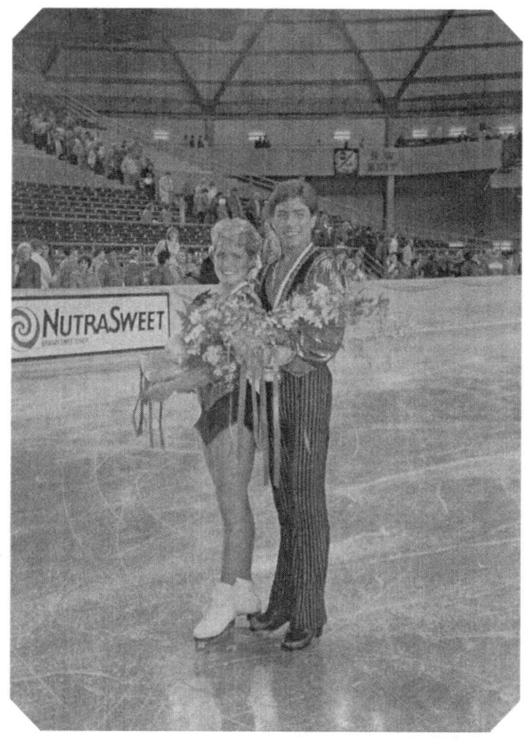

Suzy and I share a proud moment in Tacoma, Washington, after we won our first Senior National Championship.

Chapter 26

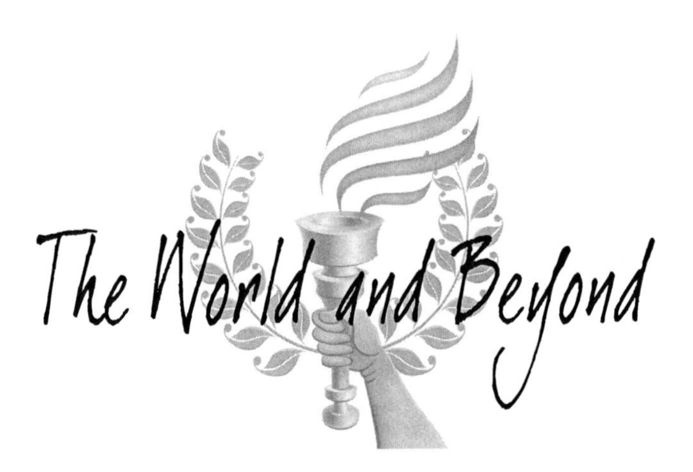

The World and Beyond

Returning to Wilmington as national champions was sweet. The glow stayed with us for several weeks; but we knew from experience that earning the title was one thing, while keeping it was another. We took some well-earned time off before we started preparing for Worlds March 10-15 in Cincinnati, Ohio.

One evening after practice, Suzy invited me to dinner at her apartment. We found ourselves revisiting the last three incredibly successful years and mulling over the possibilities for the future.

"Scott?" Suzy leaned in from the opposite side of the table. "What was it like?"

"What was what like?"

"The Olympics. What was it like to be there?"

I leaned back in the chair and laughed because I knew where she was going. "It was unlike any other competition. There's an energy charge that is so real you can almost see it. Being part of the American team is more than an honor. It's almost a sacred feeling walking in that sea of world-class athletes, knowing that you're not just skating for yourself, but for the whole nation. When Americans talk about it, they say, 'We took the gold' for a particular event. It's the scope that overwhelms you. I can't explain it, but I've tried to treat it like any other day of training. You do your run-through and try not to make any mistakes."

"I had always hoped that someday I might make it." Suzy's eyes were glistening with intensity as unshed tears promised to spill over her lower lashes.

"I didn't even think of the Olympics as a possibility until I made the decision to come to Delaware," I said, quietly putting the pieces together. "But we're close, Suzy. We're so close that nothing short of a major catastrophe could stop us."

"Don't say that!" Suzy's sharp response broke the mood.

"Say what?"

"Don't even think about catastrophes." She stood and started gathering plates from the table.

"I only meant . . ." But I could see the conversation was over. Suzy's unreasonable reaction washed over me like a cold chill. I went to the sink to dry the dishes she was feverishly washing, looking for an excuse to leave sooner than planned.

Fully psyched for Worlds, we continued to train. As national champions, we felt a greater responsibility to do well heading into Worlds. We were fifth last year, but I was convinced we could do better this year.

Before we knew it, the world competition was upon us. Even though competing in foreign countries offered certain perks, nothing compared with an international event on our own soil. Every day the arena was packed with fellow Americans who cheered us on, even during our practices. During one of our practice sessions, Suzy and I were running through one of our compulsory dances. When we finished, the Americans cheered. We waved at them as we skated to the boards to get Robbie's take on our dance.

"This is crazy," I said.

"Enjoy it, and skate for them," he replied.

We couldn't believe it! They acted like we were rock stars. Every time we would do something, there was applause. When we ran through part of our program or did a little lift, there was applause. So the practice sessions were almost like the real thing. We couldn't let our guard down, ever. It was a good five days of intense practice.

Once the competition started, we quickly established ourselves in fifth place. On the final day, we hoped our last dance would help move us up in the rankings. It may have been cold outside, but it was warm under the lights in the arena. Tension was high as we prepared to perform our free dance. Just like in Tacoma, the audience went nuts over our final presentation. We even won over a few judges, but not enough of them because we remained in fifth place. While our position in the standings was respectable, it was still rather disappointing; however, that's the world of figure skating. Our scores are subjective, so it's never a clear win as with sports like track and field events. Our judges' marks were colored by views, attitudes, and politics. But on the positive side, I was encouraged by the fact that we were obviously gaining favor with some judges. I wanted to do better so that we could have a real shot at the bronze in next year's Winter Olympics and stand in the winner's circle in my sport's pinnacle event.

It was foggy, cold, and rainy when we left Cincinnati. We were confident that the rest of the year would be awesome, and it was. We were invited to participate in the 20th Annual Tom Collins World Tour, which began three days after the close of Worlds. We flew home, washed our clothes, packed for the longer event, and then flew into Hartford, Connecticut.

They called it a "world" tour, but it was more like bringing world-class skaters into the North American arena. Mr. Collins, who preferred to be called Tommy, selected teams representing gold, silver, and bronze medal winners along with outstanding contenders in the figure skating world. We skated in a total of sixteen cities in various states, including Massachusetts, New Jersey, California, and points in between. The tour ended on April 7th, so we spent a lot of time on the road. This was a working vacation, filled with perks and opportunities to skate without competing.

Besides paying us well, Tommy made sure that we saw the sights in every major city. He took us to incredible restaurants and shows throughout the tour. It was awesome, like a great reward after a long season of hard, hard work.

Before the tour ended, Suzy and I started looking for the next season's music. After the tour, we took two weeks off to rest, relax, and prepare for our new routines. After all, 1988 was the big year—an Olympics year—and our momentum was building.

It didn't take long to find the right combination of music: a modern classical arrangement that closed with the Horace staccato, a fast-paced, high-energy trumpet piece. (We were striving for a more mature look that year.)

With our music set, our summer training went smoothly, despite my concern about some back pain issues. But this was the "no pain, no gain" era. Besides, we were on track and ready for an invitation from Harvard University's Jimmy Fund committee. Called "An Evening with Champions," this early winter event raised money for cancer research. It was initiated in 1970 by former U. S. champion John Misha Petkevich and continues to be run entirely by Harvard University students. It was a lot of fun for us to stay in the dorms with the students and share our experiences.

Even though this was an all-volunteer event, our participation not only gave us an opportunity to test our free dance number before a live audience, but the recorded program increased our exposure because it was aired on various networks throughout the year.

When we arrived in Boston, the weather was blustery and cold. Some Harvard University students met us at the airport and took us back to their respective dorms. We met for dinner and then headed to a reception where the athletes would meet faculty and guests.

Harvard is an Ivy League school that has a rich history and tradition. But college is still college, and once the formal festivities were over, our hosts took us to the Ratskeller so we could hang out and relax.

The next morning, Suzy and I met up at the rink, where we practiced for two hours and generally prepared for the night's event. When it was our time to perform, we skated like the national champions we were. The audience loved our free dance filled with new moves and lifts, which were right on the mark, and I was feeling stronger than ever. Another round of parties closed out the event, and we found ourselves on an airplane heading back to Wilmington.

A funny thing started happening during our training: the back pain that plagued me during the summer came more often, and with greater intensity. I was used to an occasional spasm, even though I was in top form, but now it was almost routine. Normally, after skating our program in full, we would skate laps around the rink as fast as we could to help increase our endurance. But now, instead of skating laps after my run-throughs, I had to hunch over to relieve the pain and skate to the side. When I could move again, I would go to the locker room, lay down with my back on the bench, and pull my knees up to stretch my muscles. Doing this for about five minutes would normally calm the spasm so I could continue to train.

One day, Robbie found me stretching in the locker room.

"Having trouble, Scott?"

"Yeah," I replied. "Same old stuff, but it seems to be getting worse."

"Better check it out."

I made an appointment to see a doctor the next day. He didn't find anything wrong with my back, yet he sent me to physical therapy to help me keep anything bad from happening. But I'd had enough of that therapy earlier in my career with my knees, and I didn't need it now. Despite my back pain, we intensified our training by adding twenty minutes of grueling stroking exercises at the end of the day.

It was mid-November, about two weeks after the Jimmy Fund event. We were scheduled for an international event in Germany. After skating a great program in Boston and feeling our momentum growing, I looked forward to this competition and the season leading up to the Olympics.

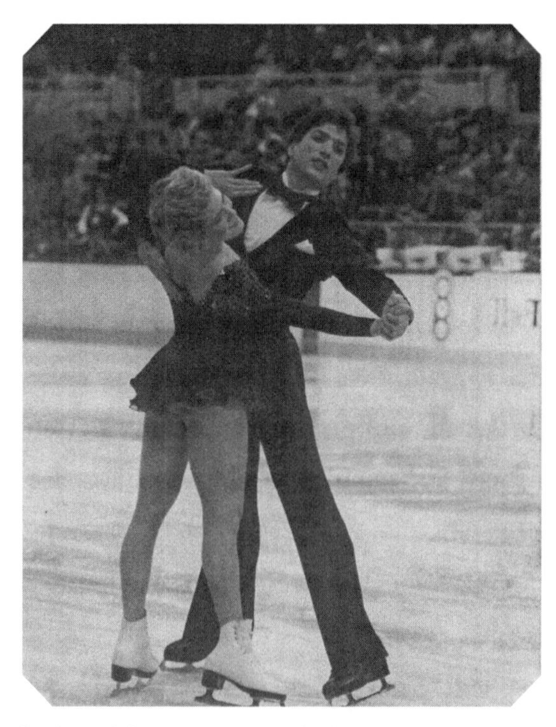

Performing with Suzy as we gear up for the next competitive season.

Chapter 27

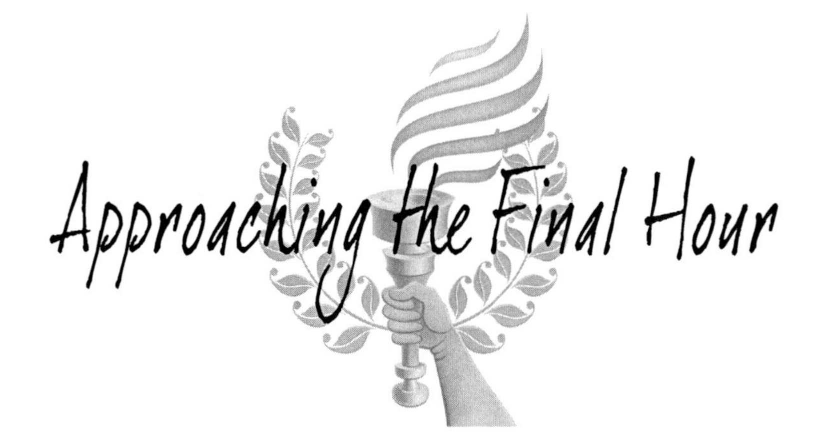

Approaching the Final Hour

The eight-hour flight to Frankfurt, Germany, seemed longer than most. I felt my back getting stiff; so I would get up, stretch, and move around as much as I could. Noticing an ever-increasing pain, I moved slowly, assuming it was just caused by the stiffness.

When we landed, I waited until most of the people were off the plane before I got up to pull my skate bag from the overhead compartment. My teammates were well ahead of me and through customs by the time I got to the check-in point.

"Your first time in Germany?" the tall, blond customs agent said as he reviewed my passport. He was all business.

"Yes," I replied, stretching my back.

"Your reason for visiting?"

"A skating competition," I replied.

"Your teammates came through here about ten minutes ago."

"Yes, sir," I replied as he returned my passport.

"Enjoy your stay in West Germany."

The pain in my back continued to bother me as I walked the length of the corridor to the conveyor belt that transferred our luggage from the handlers' trucks to the building. I carefully pulled my bag off the belt and hauled it to the bus that was waiting to take us to the hotel.

No one was very talkative because the long flight wore us out. We couldn't get to the hotel fast enough to suit me. Once the elevator took us to our floor, I found my room on the left, dropped my luggage just inside the door, and made a beeline for the bed. Lying down for the first time, I felt the tension in my back relax. I quickly fell into a deep sleep—so deep that I didn't hear my roommate, U. S. pairs skater, Peter Oppegard, arrive moments later.

Bright sunshine sneaking through the blinds, accompanied by a rumbling in my stomach, told me that I'd slept through dinner. It was morning. I sat up in bed, gently twisted my torso, and felt my usual stiffness when Peter stepped out of the bathroom, fully dressed and ready to go.

"You must have been tired," he said as he picked up his skate bag. "I've got an early practice, but they're serving breakfast for another two hours."

"Thanks," I said, swinging around to get up. "See you later."

I had the room to myself almost before I finished my sentence. This wasn't good: I didn't like starting the day so late. But after a hot shower and a good breakfast, I felt even better. Suzy and I met Robbie at the bus and rode to the rink together.

Arriving at the building, we scoped out the rink (which included finding out where the judges would sit) and got a general feel for the layout of our program. These early morning practice sessions were not well-attended, except by a few locals, family members, and some judges who liked to get an idea of pre-competition standings. Even though my parents were usually at the international events, their work schedules kept them from attending this time.

Suzy and I finished our warm-up and were ready for the run-through. The music started, and about forty seconds into the routine, we did our first lift. I bent over to grab Suzy's waist and leg. As soon as I came up and started to lift her, I felt it—an unfamiliar sensation in my back. I wasn't in pain, but I knew something bad had happened. Yet I couldn't stop, because we were trained not to stop. That was all we needed—for a judge to decide that we weren't medal material.

As we continued our program, I felt a burning that started in my lower back and traveled down my left leg. My muscles went into a spasm, tightening like a unified army moving ever forward to the mark. Then, we were finished, and the music stopped. Pain and weakness assaulted me all at once. No amount of determination could keep me standing, and I keeled over.

"Scott? What's wrong?" Suzy's expression unmasked her confusion. "Scott?"

I shook my head but couldn't speak. She wrapped her right arm around my waist and helped me skate back to Robbie.

"Scott! You're white as a sheet!" Robbie said as Suzy and I closed in on the boards.

"My back, it's my back!" My voice was more of a croak.

"Can you skate?"

"I don't know, maybe," I said trying to straighten up. "My leg isn't working. It hurts. But maybe if . . ."

Before I could finish, Robbie made the call. He knew that when I said "it hurts" that it was more than a bump in the road.

"You're done," Robbie said. "Go into the locker room and lay down. I'll meet you there."

I wouldn't have argued with him even if I could. I felt clammy and sweaty at the same time. Searing pain kept me half-bent over as Suzy bore most of my weight, while steering me back across the ice toward the locker room on the opposite side of the rink. My left leg was useless. Robbie was jogging along the perimeter to meet us on the other side.

I hurt too much to feel foolish or even care what the people in the stands or my competitors might be thinking. Robbie met us just outside the locker room and half-carried me inside. I dropped onto the first available bench, where I laid down. He removed my skates.

"What happened out there?" he asked, squatting on the floor so he could see my face.

"I don't know. I was doing my lift, and it felt like my back blew out."

"Scott?" a Japanese competitor stopped by to see how I was doing. He looked concerned. "You all right?"

"I don't know," I replied, the pain notching up a bit.

He walked away, shaking his head and muttering.

"It'll be another hour before we can get back to the hotel," Robbie continued. "Will you be all right here, or should we call for an ambulance?"

"Maybe if I rest, I'll get better," I replied.

Robbie nodded his head, patted my shoulder, and left the changing room. I didn't get better. By the time the bus arrived, I could hardly move at all. Robbie and Suzy practically carried me to it.

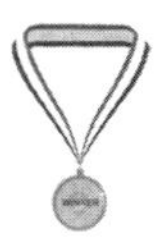

When we got back to the hotel, Robbie helped get me to my room. Peter was already there, gathering up his stuff when Robbie managed to get the door open.

"Hey, man, I heard about what happened," Peter said as he rushed to help us in.

I tried to nod my head, but every movement was agony. My left leg was beyond useless by this time.

"Sorry for your luck," he said.

"Thanks," I replied.

Then he was gone.

"Scott, I'll be back in about an hour," Robbie said, closing the curtains. "We've arranged for a car to take us to the hospital."

"Have you called my mom?" Whispers of a memory took me back to the time when I blew out my knee in Skaneateles.

"Yeah," he said. "I'm going to call her back after you see the doctors here. We've moved Peter to another room so you can rest undisturbed. We'll also be bringing your meals here. Try to rest now. I'll be back in about an hour to take you to the hospital."

"Thanks," I said, trying to push back my anger and disappointment. I closed my eyes in an attempt to block the throbbing pain in my back. Shadows of past injuries threatened to overtake me as I heard the door shut. I felt alone, abandoned, and adrift. Then my memories meandered to my recuperation back home, at the beginning of my partnership with Suzy. I remembered the peace I felt at the lake. Surely, I hadn't come this far to have it all taken away from me so abruptly. That thought comforted me as I slipped into a restless sleep.

"Scott?" Suzy's voice pulled me from the throbbing darkness.

"What?" I sounded groggier than I meant to be.

"Scott, it's time to go see the doctors."

I opened my eyes to the darkened room. I lifted my head, looking for the source of the squeaking wheels drawing closer to my bed. That single movement engaged the pain receptors in my brain. I immediately tensed and tried to consciously relax.

"Come on, Scott," Robbie said as he rolled an ancient wheelchair to my bedside.

"In that?" I wasn't sure it would hold me.

"For you, for now, it's better than walking."

Robbie gently placed his hand under my shoulder to lift me up and Suzy guided my feet over the edge of the bed. Getting into the wheelchair seemed like a major production, but we somehow managed to accomplish our goal.

"I called Dr. Angela Smith in the United States," Robbie said, as he started wheeling me toward the door. "She's already been in touch with the doctors here. They know we're coming."

Crisp, cold air surrounded me as we left the hotel and navigated into the waiting green van. They had commandeered a long, skinny vehicle so I could lay down on the trip. Taking up the whole back seat, I was vaguely aware of the scenery as we rode through the city to the hospital. Everything about Frankfurt was modern and clean, but that didn't encourage me at all. I was broken, and I didn't like it.

The more I moved, the more I hurt. By the time I was in the examining room, I could barely stand the pain. After the doctors evaluated me and took x-rays, I knew that the worst was coming. Though their English was difficult to understand, the expressions on their faces spoke volumes.

"Mr. Kaine," the lead doctor said to Robbie, "this is very bad."

"How bad?" Robbie sounded as nervous as I felt.

"He has two ruptured discs—L-4, which is here, and L-5," he said, pointing his pen to the illuminated x-ray. "We must operate immediately."

"No!" I shouted. "Not here!"

The doctor turned to me, looking quite offended.

"If we don't operate now, you will never walk again, young man. And as for skating, you're done." His lack of a bedside manner didn't bother me.

"What he means is that he would prefer to have the doctors at home work with him. They know his history," Robbie said, obviously trying to unruffle the feathers that my outburst had stirred. "Can you give him the suppositories Dr. Smith recommended? Can we just manage his pain until we get him home?"

"This is against my better judgment," the doctor replied, "but we will do as you request. Keep him off his feet. Rest is the best thing for him now."

We remained quiet on the ride back to the hotel, until we were about a block away.

"He's wrong," I said.

"About what?" Suzy sounded like she'd been crying.

"We're going to Nationals . . . and then to the Olympics." My voice sounded stronger than I felt. "I haven't come this far to quit."

Suzy looked at me. "But Scott, the doctor said—"

"Whatever it takes," I replied, determination and anger welling up within me. "I haven't come this far to be taken down like this. Keep practicing, Suzy. I'm not finished."

Suzy nodded her head and then climbed out of the car to help Robbie get me back into the wheelchair. I knew I'd been through this before—maybe not this bad, but bad enough. But I didn't have a year to give this to heal. This was my time and my shot, so I needed to be ready.

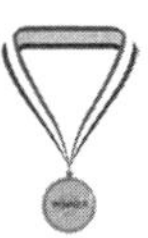

While the American team competed, I stayed in the darkened hotel room on medication designed to release the pressure on my spine. By the third day, I could walk by myself, but my leg had no feeling and my sense of balance was nil.

There were times when the entire U. S. team would gather in my room to check on me. Robbie called the doctors back home daily with progress reports. I had been down before, but not like this. I was ready to go home and work with the doctors I knew—the ones who could get me back on my feet in time for the national championships in Denver, Colorado, barely two months away.

Finally, the competition was over. We were supposed to be returning home with Robbie and Suzy in coach seating, but the United States Figure Skating Association upgraded me to first class. Robbie took care of everything, from moving my bags to briefing the airline staff about my limitations.

First class was a much different experience than coach. More leg room and seats with a longer reclining angle helped make the flight bearable. Robby, Suzy, and I boarded last.

"He's right here on the aisle," the flight attendant said as an airport staffer wheeled me to my seat.

"Don't try to help us," Robbie said as I tried to stand. Robby got behind the chair and lifted me from under the arms, while the staffer lifted me from under the knees. Pain shot through me as I struggled to remain silent. My whole body throbbed as the sharp ache radiated from my lower back. Robbie repositioned me in the seat so that my spine aligned with its contour.

"Walkman," I whispered as Suzy started to put my bag in the storage bin above me. She zipped open my bag and pulled out my tape player.

"We need some water," Robbie said, retrieving two round tablets from his coat pocket.

"What's that?" I barely recognized my own voice.

"Morphine," he said. "It will dull the pain and let you sleep."

"I hate pills," I said, as the flight attendant handed him the water.

"You need to take your seats," she said. "We'll be taking off in a few minutes."

"If you need anything, we're here," Suzy whispered in my ear. And then she was gone. I was left alone to wonder if all this work was for nothing.

"I have a blanket and some pillows for you," the flight attendant said. After plumping the pillows and fussing over me, she finally left me alone. I placed the Walkman headset over my ears and let my favorite music overtake me. Then I drifted into an almost dreamless sleep that took me through the eight-hour flight across the Atlantic and home. Totally unaware of the time passing, I reluctantly responded to the flight attendant's second call.

"Excuse me, sir, we're about to land. We have to sit you up now."

I was groggy, almost unaware of my surroundings. Pain pummeled my senses as she tried to gently raise my seat back. Only then was I aware of being in an airplane.

"A wheelchair will be waiting for you at the gate."

Robbie and Suzy got to my seat shortly before the wheelchair. We met my mother at the baggage claim area, where she took charge of me from that point on. The next day I was in Dr. Silby's office in Maryland.

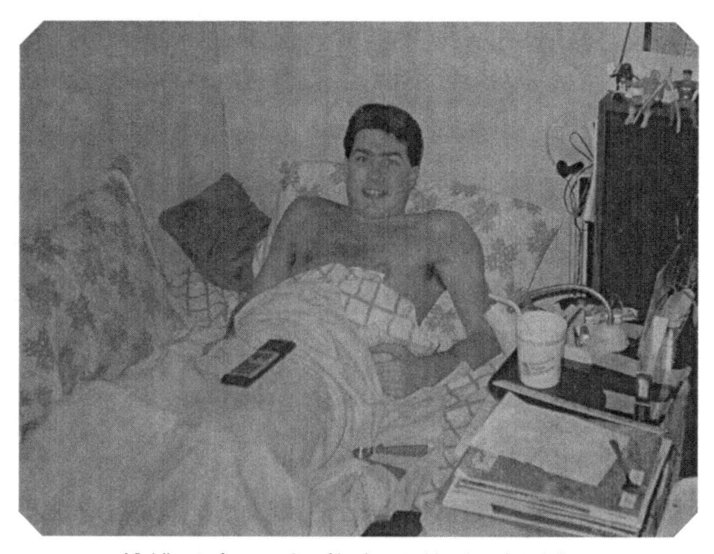

Yielding to four weeks of bed rest with a herniated disc,
I'm practicing my "champion mindset" smile through the pain.
Note the makeshift bed and good luck friend, Hulk Hogan, holding a wishbone (top right).

CHAPTER 28

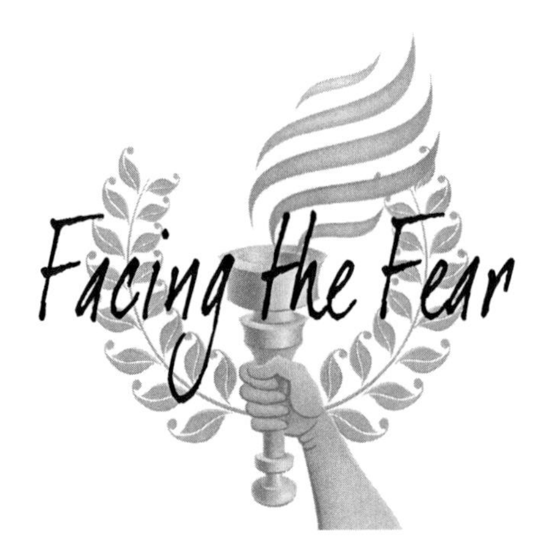

Facing the Fear

Even though the German doctors were unquestionably competent, I knew that Dr. Silby was my best option if I wanted to continue skating. I had known him for years and got to see him more often because of his participation in international events. He was well-versed in sports medicine and figure skaters' needs.

"Scott," he said, with the seriousness of my condition written all over his face, "this is the largest herniated disc I've seen in all my twenty years of practicing medicine."

"Okay," I replied, almost afraid to breathe. "So, what do we have to do?"

"Ten years ago, surgery would have been your only option."

"Two months." The catch in my throat threatened to break. "I have two months to get back on the ice and ready for Nationals."

"That's pushing it," Dr. Silby said quietly.

"Then, let's push. What do I have to do?"

"Bed rest, steroids, and a back brace, followed by physical therapy."

"How long?"

"If you're lucky, you can be back on the ice in six weeks."

I was in no mood to argue. This couldn't be happening to me—not this, not now. I refused to believe that a stupid injury would keep me from my dream when I was so close.

"I can't be off more than four weeks."

Dr. Silby just nodded his head.

I glanced up at my mother, who was standing in the corner, tight-lipped.

"What happens if he does too much too soon?" she asked. She knew me well. She knew that I went crazy when I was off my feet too long and if I rushed getting back on the ice, I could reinjure myself.

"He has a lot going for him—he's an athlete in top physical condition. I think we can get him up and on his feet for Nationals. After that, we'll see. Surgery isn't out of the picture."

She nodded her head quietly and stepped out of the exam room while I got ready to face the outside world once again. Mom and Dad both stayed with me during the worst of it; in fact, their presence made it more bearable.

The next three weeks were sheer torment. I was surprised by the number of people who came by on a regular basis to visit and keep me from going nuts. Much to my surprise, Lisa was one of the first. She was doing well in college and was planning to get married soon. She looked happy.

Todd, my mom, and my other housemates were great. They moved me to the ground floor, where it would be easier to take care of the necessities. We made a little bedroom in the den. I had a tray table set up beside me for things like TV remotes, water, pens, pencils, paper, and videotapes of Suzy and me. If I couldn't be on the ice, at least I could review our recorded practice sessions and keep them fresh in my mind.

A physical therapist came by for about two weeks to exercise the muscles in my legs and feet, keeping them toned and shaped. Since the last thing I needed was for atrophy to set in, he showed my mother how to help me continue the exercises in his absence.

One of the worst parts of my recovery period involved steroids, which I hated. When I was on them, a stranger seemed to live inside of me. I didn't like the person that these drugs made me. I'd get angry for no reason at all. The worst came out around Thanksgiving when my dad watched the Sycracuse Orangemen basketball team's televised game. The constant thudding of the ball and raucous cheering of the crowd started getting on my nerves.

"Dad, change the channel," I said.

Pound, pound, whoosh, cheer.

"Dad, change it, now!" My exploding anger surprised even me.

"Scott?" Mom said as entered the room.

Dad just ignored me.

"It's that, that stupid—"

"Scott, isn't it time for your stretches?"

I sat fuming for a moment and then nodded in agreement while Mom turned down the television and started working with me. I don't know how anyone could take these drugs if they didn't have to.

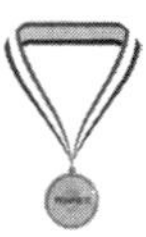

All the while, Suzy kept practicing without me. Our friend, Jeff DiGregorio, who was one of Luddy's skaters, worked with her on endurance stroking. This helped keep her motivated, in shape, and moving forward. Lord knows that she would have to be in great shape to carry me through when I got back on the ice.

After four weeks of this enforced rest period, the doctors said I could get out of my makeshift bed and start a restricted training schedule. Suzy picked me up at the house and took me to the rink.

The closer we got to the building, the faster my heart started pounding.

"You're sure you're ready for this?" Suzy sounded concerned.

"I'm ready." My voice sounded more confident than I felt. But all feelings aside, I was happy to be out of the den, despite my body's shortcomings.

Suzy stopped the car and was out before I could open my door.

"Let me help you," she said as she pulled the door open with my hand already on the inside handle. She caught me as I almost fell out.

"I'm not made of glass!" I grumbled. "If I can't get myself out of a car, how do you expect me to skate?"

"I'm sorry!" Suzy sniped back. "I'm just trying to help. I don't know what to do!"

My frustration gave way to regret. Of course she didn't know; neither did I.

"It's not your fault," I mumbled, straightening my stiff body as I got out of the car.

Slowly, I walked to the rink and followed the familiar path to the locker room where I changed clothes and put on my skates. A hush fell over the rink as I walked by, but I barely noticed. The brisk air of the artificially cooled rink was a sweet aroma to my senses, blocking out all but the best memories. Crossing the threshold, I dropped the bag in front of my locker and started getting ready for my five minutes on ice.

My absence heightened the anticipation. As I laced up my skates, left foot first, then right, my heart started pounding like a kid in a candy store getting ready to pick out my favorite. I smiled for the first time in weeks, a real smile. Minutes later, I was by the ice.

It was a typical day at the rink, filled with Luddy's teams working with their coaches. Those who knew me well appeared to be fully focused on their work until Robbie and I got on the ice. Then they stopped and watched, waiting to see how I would do.

My body wasn't working the way it had before. I knew how to skate in my mind, but my body acted like it had never been there before. My weakened ankles bowed out like some cowboy who'd been riding the range too long, so I was shaky—way too shaky.

I had no sense of feeling in my left foot. The ruptured disc had severed some nerves, so my left leg was not receiving messages from my brain. The tactile feelings that governed my movements were gone. This shut-down was new to me, unfamiliar, and more than uncomfortable. Becoming accustomed to this new perception of skating with all its nuances such as edges, leaning, and balance made me feel like a baby taking his first step.

"I'll be right behind you," Robbie said. "We only have five minutes, so let's make the most of it. Do you have any feeling in your left leg at all?"

I shook my head no, fighting to relax and dismiss the anger that threatened to break loose.

"Okay, then you'll have to measure your movements by sight."

"What?"

"By sight, like your dad does when he flies and the radar's out."

"What do you mean?"

"You're going to use your eyes to judge your position. Let's give it a try, just once around. I'll be behind you, telling you which way to lean. You'll adjust and learn when you're on the mark by what and how you see. This will work. Trust me."

I stroked out to the right on my strong leg and then shifted to my left, but it wouldn't hold my weight and slipped out from underneath me. Robbie grabbed me as I started to fall. Straightening up, I saw my friends turn quickly away, like they didn't want me to know they had seen.

"Don't look at them," Robbie growled. "Focus on what we're doing."

Focusing straight ahead, I re-ordered my mind and repeated the exercise. This time I was ready for the stroke and was prepared for its lazy route forward. Instead of falling, I tried to compensate by adjusting my weight in. It was like trying to walk on a leg that has fallen asleep. It's there, but you're just not sure where.

"Good," Robbie said, "lean a bit more to the left."

Slowly, we worked our way around the rink. This time, I barely noticed the faces of skaters who had once looked up to me and applauded my skill. Even with a cursory glance, it was obvious that they didn't think I'd make it back. By the time my five minutes were up, I felt like I'd worked out all day. It was hard, almost too hard. Breathing heavily and starting to break a sweat, I leaned on Robbie as he helped me back into the changing room.

"Scott, do you need help removing your skates?"

"I can do it myself." I stopped my complaint that threatened to erupt when I saw Luddy standing in the doorway. Without saying a word, he nodded his head briskly and then turned and left. I looked at Robbie.

"They don't think I can do this, do they?" I ask, yielding to the doubts that harassed me.

"What they think doesn't matter," he said.

"Yeah, but why didn't Luddy say anything?"

"Because he didn't have to."

"What do you mean?"

"Do you think he'd let you come back if he didn't know you could do this?"

I couldn't reply. I could only shake my head, but I didn't feel much better.

I was so angry by the time I got home, all I could do was beat my bed with my fists. My greatest enemy was doubt, which was eroding my confidence level. It was less than a month away from Nationals, and I couldn't even skate around the rink once! Five minutes took all the energy and strength I had, and I was worse than bad.

But Robbie was right to encourage me. I went back to the rink the next day and skated for ten minutes. Every muscle in my body ached from the previous day's workout. It hurt, but I had to do this.

I was allowed to increase my session time by five minutes a day. Mid-week I skated with Suzy. Robbie and Luddy stood at the boards, watching us closely.

Suzy took my hand, and together we navigated the circumference of the rink, with neither of us saying a word. My whole body was shaking, while my mind's voice repeated every action over and over. We finished at our point of departure, by Robbie and Luddy.

"You did fine, Scott," Luddy said, his voice more encouraging than his demeanor.

I looked at Suzy. Silent tears had left soft streaks on her cheeks. In fact, she was a mess by the end of the session. Frustration welled up in me. I didn't want pity! I wanted my body to work the way it had before!

It took a week to work up to thirty-minute sessions. My second week on the ice was a little more promising. We started working on our dances, progressing at a snail's pace. By the end of the week, we started running through the programs a little faster and pushed them out a little more. I still had no feeling in my left leg, which remained stiff. Thankfully, however, my right leg worked just fine.

On and off the ice, I felt insecure and out of place, like I was letting people down. I was progressing, but not fast enough. I couldn't get through a simple pattern without stopping, because fatigue assaulted my left limb. Our dance was junk. Skating like a beginner, I knew I was holding Suzy back.

Once back at the house, I got into a major fight with myself. With my confidence shaken, I knew we needed a break—a real miracle that would release us to go to the Olympics, even if I couldn't skate the way I did before. It was only fair, wasn't it? It's not like I'd lost my talent. I just needed a little more time, that's all. That wasn't too much to ask, was it?

The clock was ticking. Grasping for a miracle, I thought that maybe as the current national champion who was fifth in the world rankings, I could bypass Nationals and go straight to the Olympics.

I picked up the phone to call a top official. Explaining my predicament, I held my breath until he responded.

"I heard you got hurt," he said, "but what you're asking is not possible." The immovable wall on the other side sucked the last glimmer of hope from my soul.

"I see," I said, trying to keep my trembling voice from screaming. "I'm just not sure I can be ready in time."

The voice softened. "I wish I could help you, Scott, but I can't. It's not what you've done in the past that counts. It's what you can do now. Good luck."

"Okay." A sad, weak breath escaped from my tightened chest. "I'll see you in Denver."

The moment I replaced the phone handset in its cradle, I broke down. My positive attitude shifted into reverse as I fell to my knees and started screaming.

"Why? Why?" I yelled. I was alone in the house. This was between God and me.

"Why did You let this happen? I need Your help so much, but where are You? Why haven't You healed me fast enough? Did You bring me this far to drop me? I don't understand! I need You now!"

I continued wailing for five minutes or so until I noticed the last beam of sunshine peeking through my window, drawing my attention to the view on the other side. As I pulled my focus from myself and started toward the window, a slight change inched its way into my spirit. Unsteadily, I crawled to the aperture. Grasping the sill, I pulled myself up. My gaze settled on the world around me—people coming home from work and children greeting their parents. This was a scene being replayed in homes throughout America. With dusk rapidly approaching, my internal view shifted as well.

I have to do this. I can do this. I will beat this. I'm going to do this, just wait and see. Then a foreign peace descended upon me. Weary and emotionally spent, I lay down on my bed. Moments later, I was asleep.

Nothing seemed to change much during the next week. My parents came to visit for the holidays and drove me to the rink on Christmas Day. Suzy and I had scheduled an afternoon practice, and Robbie was there too.

"Come on, Scott, push through," Robbie called to us across the empty rink. Suzy and I managed to finish three-quarters of our program without stopping.

"You'll be fine," Robbie said after we finished. "You look good." I could only nod my head. I was breathing too heavily to say anything. Despite my silence, I felt good about myself and my chances; we were almost there. I couldn't have received a better Christmas present.

Robbie always made me feel better about myself, especially then. He looked for the positive and helped me build on it, but he was that way with everyone. It was a great quality in his training style.

"I'm glad you weren't here to see Scott on his first day back," Robbie said to my mom and dad.

"We figured it would be rough," Dad replied. I looked at Mom, who had tears in her eyes.

During the final week before Nationals, I struggled to get through our whole program once without stopping. Our modified routine minimized the lifts and relied heavily on energy and footwork. Since building up stamina was the key, I practiced with a scarf over my nose and mouth to duplicate the thinner air we would face in Denver, but that wasn't enough. I was normally too winded by the end of the program. I needed to do more, prepare more, and extend my energy envelope. I attacked the problem with more intense daily work-outs on my slide board at home.

The day before we left Wilmington, I managed to get through our whole program once. I could sense that my strategy worked because I had more stamina, which gave me a glimmer of hope. It was like God had given me a gift, a nod that said we would be all right. Maybe we did have a chance.

Ready or not, it was time to leave—to find out if I had recovered enough to get on the Olympic team.

Chapter 29

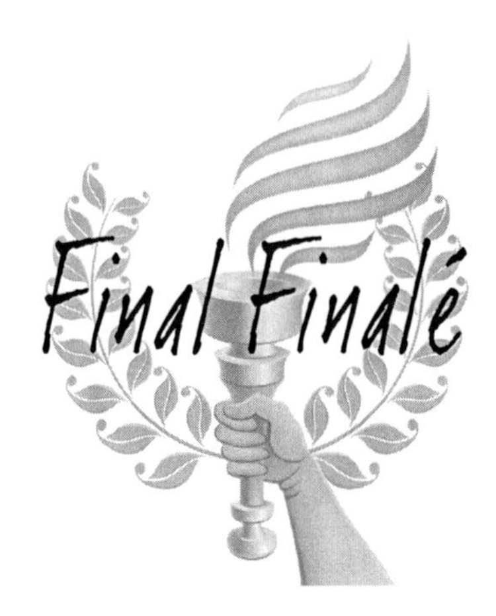

Final Finalé

Fatigue was my greatest enemy, followed closely by a leg that felt half useless. My muscles ached with each practice, and stamina seemed like a memory from another lifetime. By the time we left Wilmington for Denver, I had no idea how I would get through competition week, let alone three compulsories, our original dance, free dance, and all the practice sessions. That was my concern. That was my Achilles' heel.

Denver in January is cold, but plummeting temperatures were the least of my concerns. Under the best circumstances, competing at Nationals was stressful on multiple levels. It was mentally stressful because you had to be at the top of your form, both on the ice and off. It was physically stressful, especially in Denver, where the air was so much thinner than at home. And then there was the injury. My mind kept replaying my first five minutes back on the ice when I looked so inept and foolish, just one month ago. What was I doing here? This emotional stew started simmering the moment we stepped off the plane and continued on our drive to the hotel.

My parents insisted on renting a car so we could travel to and from the rink on our own schedule. My pride wanted to refuse their offer, but my practical side accepted this one concession to my condition. It helped a lot. Removing the anxiety of bus schedules and hurrying up to wait lightened the load a bit. It also gave me some extra time to rest between our practice sessions. I didn't need to be around other distractions, so it seemed logical. My parents were right.

After many days of stressful practice, the competition was upon us. Once at the arena, Suzy bounded out of the car. She was ready to get where she was going, fast.

"Come on, Scott," she said, almost dancing in circles.

"Go ahead," I said, moving a little slower. My stiff muscles were taking a bit longer to loosen up. "I'll meet you inside."

She stopped short and settled down a bit. "No, I'll stay with you," she said quietly. "We're a team."

Mom walked inside with us while Dad parked the car. None of us said anything. What was there to say? Once inside, we started to go our separate ways.

"Suzy, I'd like a minute with Scott," Mom looked serious, almost too serious.

"Sure, Bayne," she said. "I'll start warming up." I watched my partner walk toward an area in which we would stretch and loosen up before changing into our outfits.

Mom turned to me and gave me a hug.

"Do you have any idea of how proud we are of you?" I saw tears brimming in her eyes. All I could do was smile.

"Just go out and do your best. You do look great out there."

"Mom, I've got to go." I hugged her again and turned toward the warm-up area. I stopped for a moment and looked back. Mom was going to her seat.

Every year, compulsories are held in the main arena, but this year was different because we were in a smaller hockey-style rink. After our off-ice warm-up, Suzy and I changed clothes, put on our skates, and walked to the rink. We met Robbie and Luddy at the door leading to the ice and walked in together, knowing that the whole skating world knew of my disability and would be watching me closely.

Our first compulsory was a Tango Romantica, a stamina-rich dance that would set the pace for the rest of the competition. The music started. Totally focused on the task at hand, I willed my body to comply, and it did. Unaware of scores, standings, and the audience, I forced aching muscles to move, an uncommunicative foot to obey, and immobilizing fatigue to wait for just another stroke, just another movement. If effort was the measurement here, the required two minute routine might as well have been two hours. Suddenly the music stopped, my eternity ended, and we were finished. We took our bows and started skating toward the boards. I couldn't get to the bench fast enough. I needed to sit, rest, and recover. At the same time, I was exhilarated. I had gotten through the first dance. If I got through that one, then I knew I could get through the rest.

"Are you okay?" Suzy asked as I slumped to my seat.

I was out of breath. All I could do was nod my head. Then our scores were posted.

"Oh, my God!" Suzy almost screamed.

I looked up, and, like Suzy, I could hardly believe my eyes. Our scores were high 5's out of a perfect 6.0—we had received first-place scores for that dance. We had a real shot at holding onto the title! All I could do was smile, but that was enough.

While Suzy, Robbie, and Luddy stayed to watch the other competitors, I needed to take a break. I went out to the rental car to lie down and rest in the back seat. As I felt my muscles relax, I found myself revisiting my performance. It was absolutely unbelievable. Possibilities and hope started to push back my despair. That's when I first started believing that maybe, just maybe, my injury wouldn't hold us back.

By the end of the evening, Suzy and I had successfully completed two more compulsory dances. We kept our solid lead, but I was beginning to feel the stress in every area of my body. I was exhausted, and the thin air was getting to me. Longer periods on the ice were taking their toll. I hoped a good night's sleep would be enough to give me a fresh start the next day.

I didn't realize how taxing the first day was until we were doing our Original Set Pattern on day two. It was an intense dance. The familiar notes of our second tango filled the arena, signaling us to begin. All went well until the final quarter of the number as fatigue intruded. The

Morzine official would have been proud at this moment because of the lesson I learned. I pushed through. I didn't get this far by caving in at the first sign of resistance, so I pushed harder. The harder I pushed, the more fatigue gained momentum. Like a drowning swimmer grabbing hold of a lifesaver, I mentally grabbed the final bars of the music and forced my left leg to lift as we rounded the corner for the finish. I didn't dare breathe until after we took our bow and started skating back to the entrance. As we approached the doorway, I stepped off the ice and my left leg gave way. I almost lost my balance, but Robbie grabbed me and kept me from falling.

I laughed. "It was clean, wasn't it?"

Robbie glanced over my shoulder. "Check the scores."

Still holding onto him, I turned and looked. I wasn't sure how I could feel so miserable and so happy at the same time, but I did. We were still in first place.

Each day dragged on in slow motion, with the third day being the slowest. We would awaken in the morning and suffer through eight hours or more of anticipating that evening's competition. Successfully overcoming each obstacle added to the stress and pressure of that final day. Mentally, I was drained; I needed it to be over. The final test was the hardest, not only because it was longer and more demanding than any of the other routines, but now everyone's expectations were higher because I had gotten this far in my condition. In fact, many people told me I was looking great. They didn't notice that I had any problems at all, but they weren't in my head or my body. I couldn't see what they saw, so I assumed they were lying.

I mentally wobbled when I thought about how unprepared I was. With only one successful free dance run-through, I was supposed to compete at the national level. That went against everything I knew about being a champion. Sure, we had removed the difficult lifts and kept those that didn't strain my lower back, but I was beginning to wonder if that was enough. However, there wasn't anything else we could have done to lighten the load.

Finally, the day merged into evening, and it was time to return to the rink. My hands shook as I changed into my costume. Hoping beyond hope that this would be the right moment, I laced my skates, left foot first, then right. Suddenly, I noticed that my hands were still. I was ready. I knew I could do this.

Warm lights, cold ice, and a packed house exuded finality as we took our place center ice. Just before the spotlight surrounded us, I took a deep breath and put my arms around Suzie for our starting position. Feeling my heart pump like a turbine engine repaired many times over, my body twitched when the music began. We were in full motion, executing the modified movements that we had practiced. Step by step, I reviewed my progress while we continued. Suzy was always there, right on point. But the mental, physical and emotional strain was pushing harder to unravel me. *Push, push, push. It's only four minutes. I can do this for four minutes*—this overriding thought kept propelling me to the end. I was aware of every second eating into the routine until seconds rolled into minutes and minutes into the finalé. I felt like I was about to burst when the final notes brought us to our finish.

Shaking all over, I turned to Suzy to hug her. Suddenly, in its final act of rebellion, my leg gave way, and I collapsed to my knee, right in front of everyone. *It's done!* My mind's voice shouted. *We finished, and now I have to stand up.* Suzy helped me rise so we could finish taking our bows. Leaning on her, we returned to the kiss-and-cry area.

"Unbelievable." Robbie's voice was soft and reassuring. "You did it. You looked great."

Luddy quietly followed with a pat on my shoulder that conveyed his approval as well. That gesture said far more than any words could.

I nodded my head in agreement. *But was it enough?* Breathing heavily, I slumped onto the bench and leaned forward, with my elbows on my knees. Sweat rolled off my face as I waited for our results, too tired to care.

"Scott! Look!" Suzy's shrieking diverted my attention to the scoreboard, but it was Robbie's laughter that helped me shake off the chains of exhaustion. I looked up and saw the numbers up on the scoreboard: we won! I could barely process it.

Adrenaline replaced fatigue as we started hugging and patting each other on the back. I don't know who was more ecstatic—Robbie or Suzy. Even Luddy was more animated than usual. A week earlier and we would have been denied any chance of being national champions again. But, here we stood, a true miracle.

Moments later, we were called to take the ice as the 1988 National Ice Dance Champions. Sheer joy surrounded me as Suzy and I took our places at the top of the podium. Amazed, I looked out at the crowd. When so many others would have quit because of what could have happened, I was able to overcome the doubts to achieve something special, something outstanding, something few stay around long enough to finish. It was a simple case of persevering, no matter what stood in my way. Oddly enough, I think the judges and the audience knew that too. It was this realization, along with the joyful thought that I would return to the Olympics, that made this second championship even more memorable.

Once the ceremonies were over, the top three teams were taken to the press room. By this time, I was familiar with some of the reporters who surrounded us, asking their questions.

"Scott, after your injury, why did you come back?" one reporter asked.

"What?" I was stunned. "Uh, it never occurred to me not to."

"You almost collapsed at the end of your free dance. Wouldn't it have been easier to just quit and retire?"

"I've been training for this just about all my life. The injury was unfortunate, but I couldn't let it stop me when I had a chance to be on the Olympic team again. This is what we've worked for the last four years. I just had to give it my best, injury and all."

I saw other reporters writing fast and furiously. "I never really thought that I'd done anything special, although I dealt with ideas of quitting years ago. I didn't even think in terms of options. I believed in what I was doing, so I set my goals high. I counted on my training, determination, and drive to take care of the rest."

Returning to Delaware as national champions was sweet victory, especially for those who saw my first five minutes on the ice a month earlier. While I was preparing for Nationals, I didn't consider the broader implications of this phase of my journey. A letter from my mother helped put it all in perspective:

Jan 20, 1988

Dear Scott,

Words cannot describe the feelings Dad and I have for your strength, strong will, strong desire, guts, faith, and positive attitude. Who did you get these wonderful traits from? We truly put you on a pedestal as do so many, many other skaters, pros, judges, and people in general. You are a very special breed.

I am sure you know how heartbroken we were to hear of your mishap, but it was you with your positive attitude and "up-ness" that gave us the strength to get through this. What a wonderful character and outlook on life you have had, not only on this occasion but always. You certainly have had a lot of stumbling stones along the way, but each one has made you a stronger person. You are going to have so much to offer your children someday and those you teach or come in contact with.

When you and Suzy finished your free dance, we were so proud, more than ever before. This was such a big victory for you. It was just amazing. You had to have felt so proud of yourself. Someday I would love to know what your inner thoughts have been and how you thought you could do it. You seriously should be jotting down notes and thoughts to write a book someday. I am sure it would help many.

> Scott, you have made us extremely proud parents, not only because of your skating, but just because you are the person you are.
>
> All our love,
> Mom and Dad

My mother's letter helped me maintain my perspective while we prepared for the Olympics. My injury seemed to get as much or more attention than our second year as national champions.

Suzy and I spent the next month training for the Olympics. As my back grew stronger, we reintegrated most of the original lifts into our routine, even though I was still wearing a back brace. Though I had improved significantly, I wasn't comfortable when we reached Calgary because I had yet to regain my full strength. Because of an unfortunate misstep that might have been avoided if I'd had full feeling back in my foot, we came in sixth. But that was all right. I knew that I had done my best and had overcome insurmountable odds to achieve the goals set in front of me.

After the 1988 Olympics, Suzy continued her amateur career while I took the necessary time off for back surgery at the doctors' strong recommendation. At the age of twenty-eight, I knew that it was time to stop competing. My body had been through enough, so this part of my journey was over. It was time to leave the grueling grind of competitive skating to others who were waiting for their shot.

I returned to the University of Delaware Training Center as one of Luddy's coaches. That's where I met and and later married Pam Duane

Gregory, a fellow skater and world-renowned coach. Our daughter Victoria enjoys dance, but not necessarily on the ice. Of course, she is quite talented in many other areas and is our pride and joy.

This has been, and continues to be, a journey of many twists and turns. But I've learned through the years that things happen for a reason.

I was never alone through any of the trials. My family, friends, and God never left me or denied me. Instead, they strengthened and encouraged me, regardless of how impossible things appeared. But they were only part of the winning combination I needed to succeed. Somewhere along the line, I developed a "champion mindset" of courage and fortitude. In the end, the key to living my dream came from within. My job was to make a choice, to do my best, to keep a positive attitude, and to commit to persevere.

This is the stuff champions are made of. Do you have it in you?

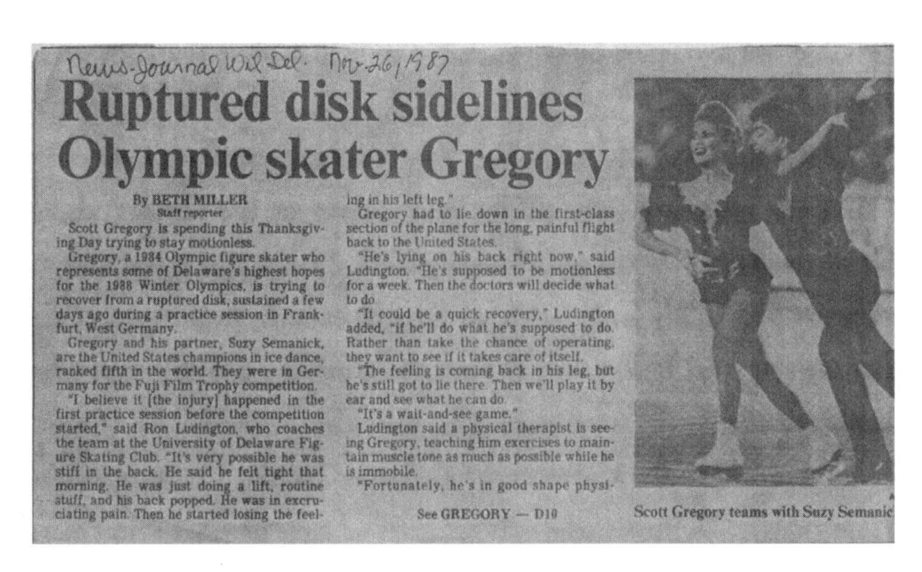

News-Journal Wil Del. Nov. 26, 1987

Ruptured disk sidelines Olympic skater Gregory

By BETH MILLER
Staff reporter

Scott Gregory is spending this Thanksgiving Day trying to stay motionless.

Gregory, a 1984 Olympic figure skater who represents some of Delaware's highest hopes for the 1988 Winter Olympics, is trying to recover from a ruptured disk, sustained a few days ago during a practice session in Frankfurt, West Germany.

Gregory and his partner, Suzy Semanick, are the United States champions in ice dance, ranked fifth in the world. They were in Germany for the Fuji Film Trophy competition.

"I believe it [the injury] happened in the first practice session before the competition started," said Ron Ludington, who coaches the team at the University of Delaware Figure Skating Club. "It's very possible he was stiff in the back. He said he felt tight that morning. He was just doing a lift, routine stuff, and his back popped. He was in excruciating pain. Then he started losing the feeling in his left leg."

Gregory had to lie down in the first-class section of the plane for the long, painful flight back to the United States.

"He's lying on his back right now," said Ludington. "He's supposed to be motionless for a week. Then the doctors will decide what to do.

"It could be a quick recovery," Ludington added, "if he'll do what he's supposed to do. Rather than take the chance of operating, they want to see if it takes care of itself.

"The feeling is coming back in his leg, but he's still got to lie there. Then we'll play it by ear and see what he can do.

"It's a wait-and-see game."

Ludington said a physical therapist is seeing Gregory, teaching him exercises to maintain muscle tone as much as possible while he is immobile.

"Fortunately, he's in good shape physi-

See GREGORY — D10

Scott Gregory teams with Suzy Semanic

My Challenge to You

I challenge you to make a choice, to keep a positive attitude no matter what negative things are thrown your way, and to be committed to persevere.

> Success is failure turned inside out—
> The silver tint of the clouds of doubt,
> And you never can tell how close you are,
> It may be near when it seems so far,
> So stick to the fight when you're hardest hit—
> It's when things seem worst that you must not quit.

Last stanza of the inspirational poem
Don't Quit by Edgar A. Guest

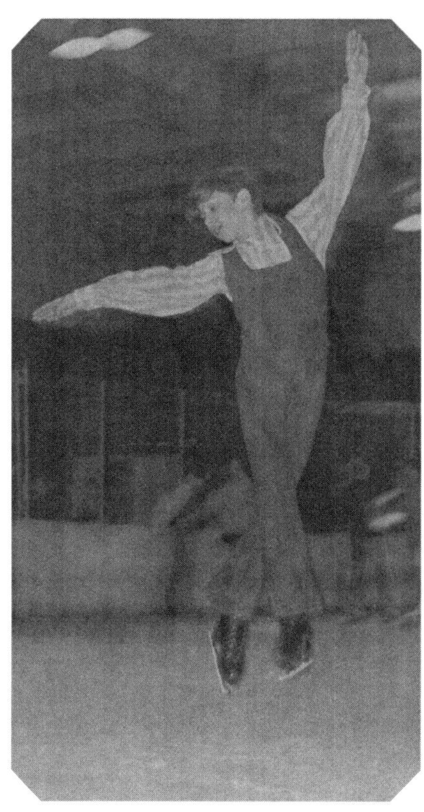

I'm showing off my mazurka at the Skaneateles Figure Skating Club. I always loved to jump as high as I could!

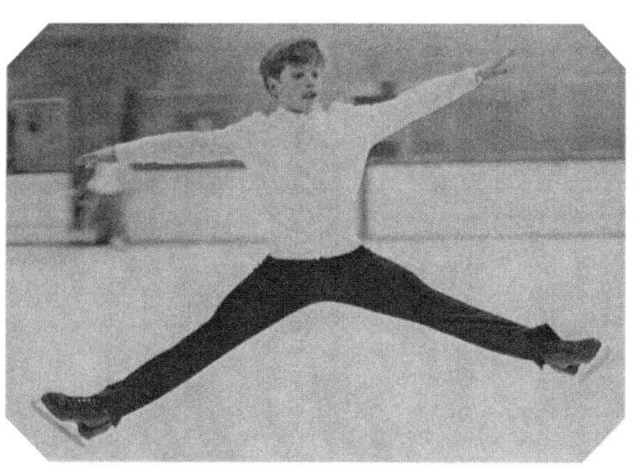

Working on my split jump
at the Skaneateles Figure Skating Club.

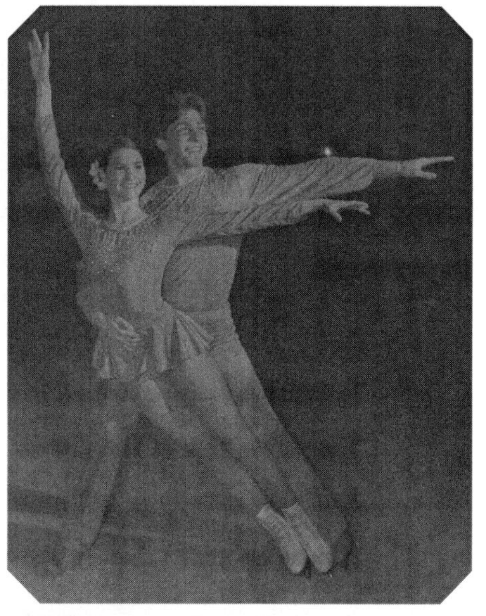

Posing for the camera with Judy
after winning Nationals in 1978.

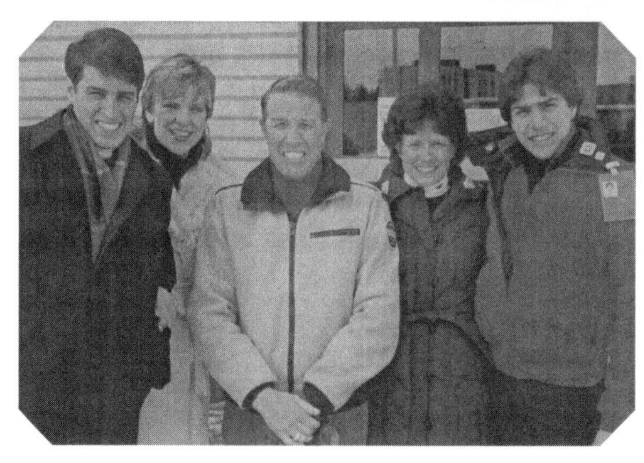

Left to right: My brother BeeGee (Bill), his wife Sharon, Dad, Mom, and me sharing a happy moment at Worlds 1982 in Copenhagen, Denmark.

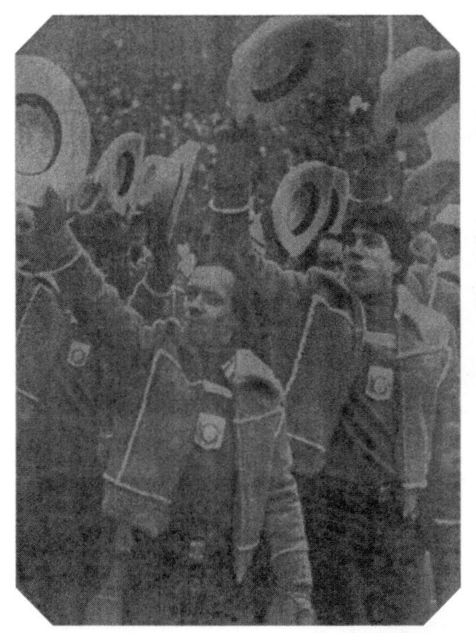

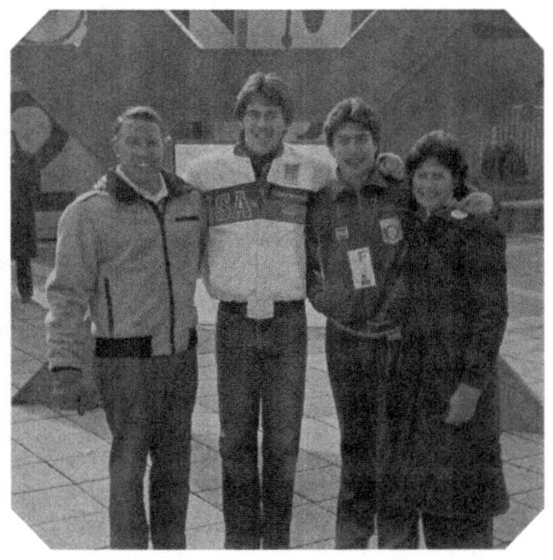

Left to right: Dad, Peter Carruthers, me, and Mom, soaking up the excitement at the Olympic Village in Sarajevo, Yugoslavia, in 1984.

Marching in the opening ceremonies in the 1984 Olympics in Sarajevo, Yugoslavia, next to Scott Hamilton–one of my most memorable moments.

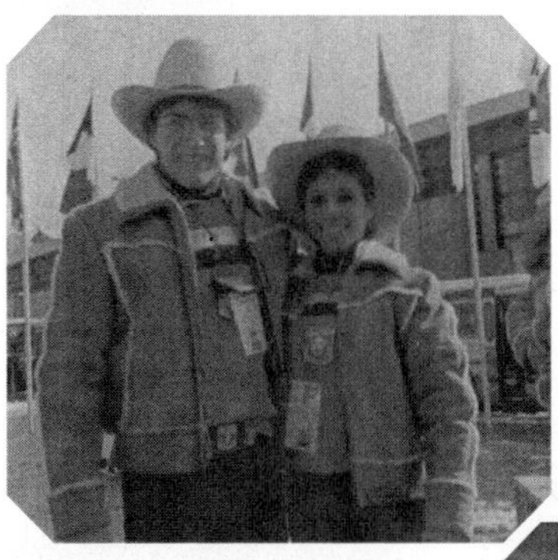

Sharing the excitement with Lisa in the Olympic Village as we prepare for the big opening ceremonies march.

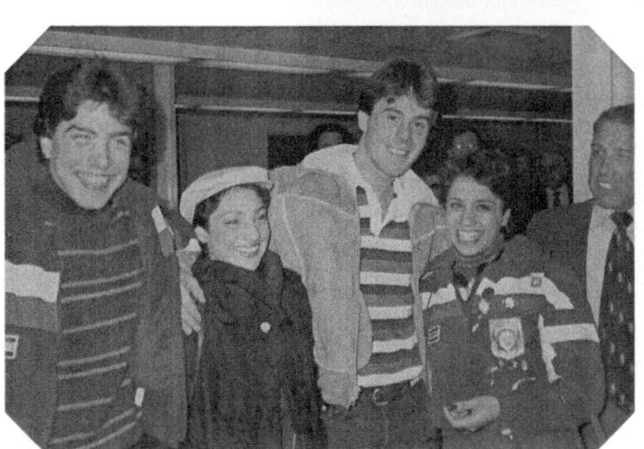

Left to right: Me, Kitty and Peter Carrothers, Lisa, and my dad, enjoying the surprise party at Skaneateles rink for the Skaneateles show in 1984.

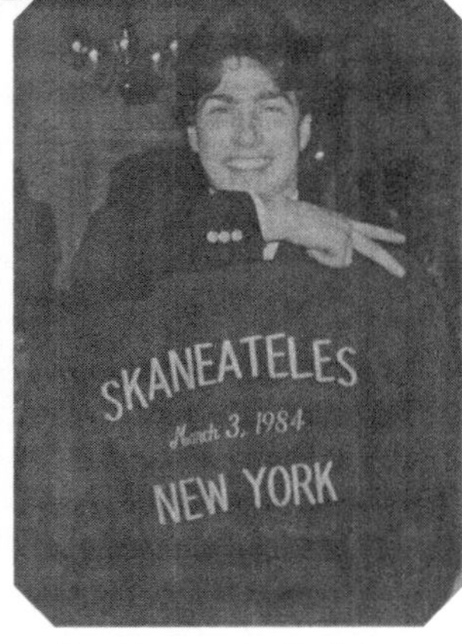

Receiving my school jacket on *Scott Gregory Day.*

Left to right: Helene Gephart ("Lady"), me, Dad, Mom, my sister Heather, her husband Jim, celebrating outside the rink at Worlds in 1986 in Cincinnati.

Skating
APRIL 1987

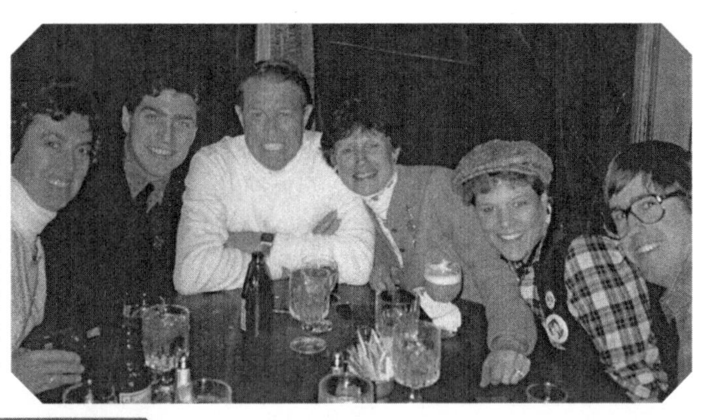

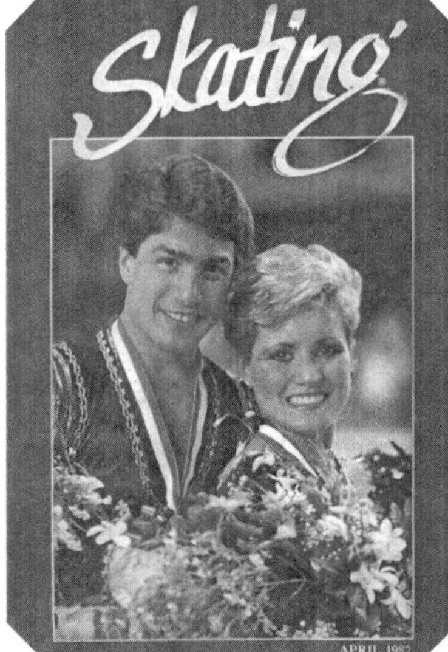

Suzy and I on the cover of *Skating* magazine after winning Nationals in 1987.

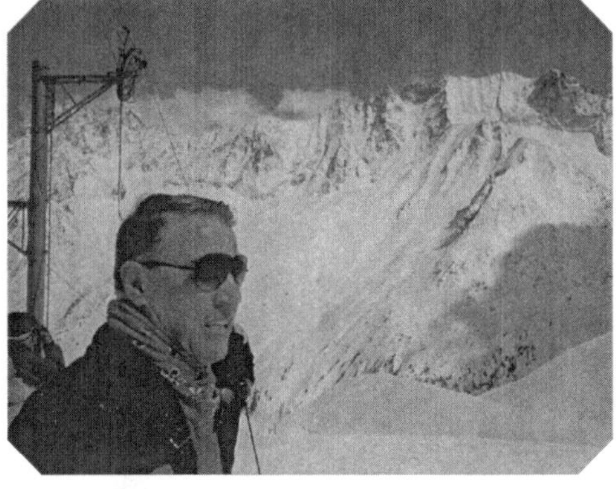

My dad enjoying the beautiful view while skiing in Arola, Switzerland, in 1987.

4 UD skaters win spots on world team

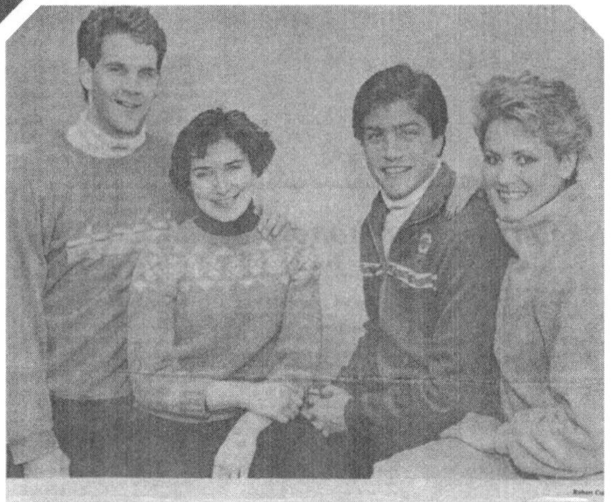

My good friend, Todd Waggoner & Gillian Wachsman (silver medalist in pairs), with Suzy and I, after winning 1987 Nationals. This photo by Robert Cohen was featured in a *News Journal* article that quoted me as saying, "I'm on cloud 10!"

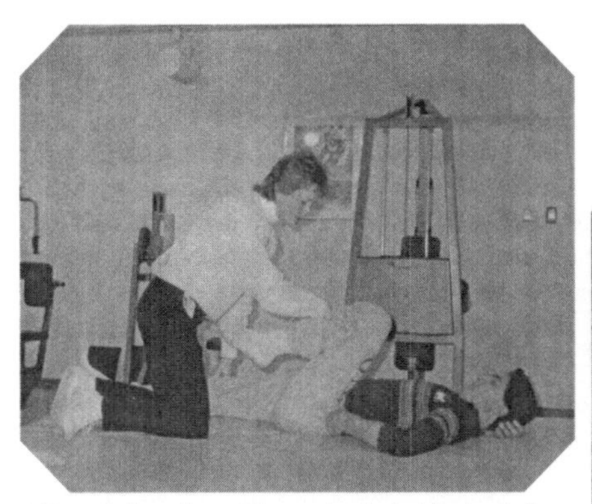

At the rehab center, getting my back stretched out after my ruptured disk, preparing for the 1988 Nationals.

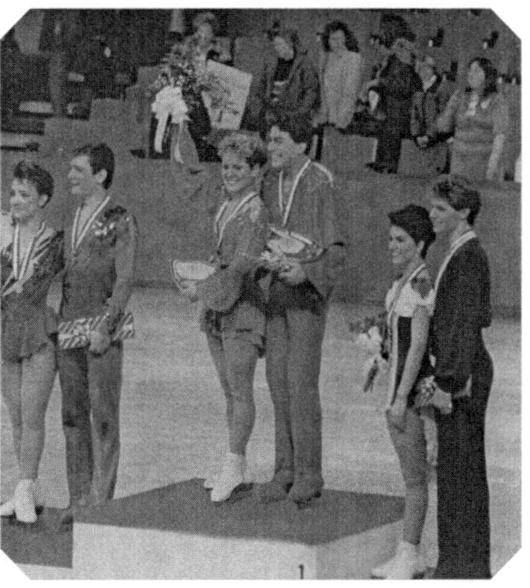

Left to right: Susan Wynne & Joe Druar (silver), Suzy & I (gold), April Sargent & Rusty Witherby (bronze) in the winners' circle at the 1988 National Championships. The expression on my face shows the mixture of relief and the overwhelming joy I was feeling.

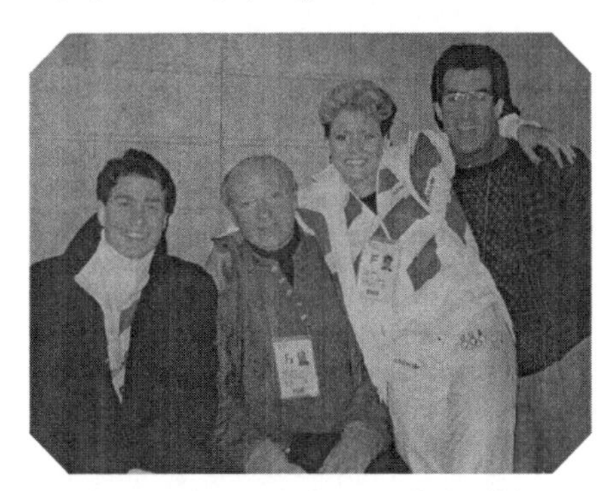

Left to right: Me, Luddy, Suzy, and Robby Kaine at the 1988 Olympics, chilling after our practice session at the competition rink in Calgary.

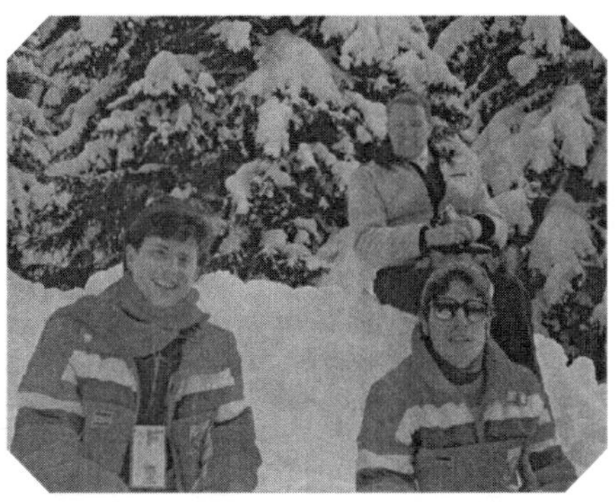

Brian Boitano and I are dressed in our Olympic jackets, watching the ski jumping event at the 1988 Olympics in Calgary. Don't miss Dad in the background, trying to blend in with the snowy trees.

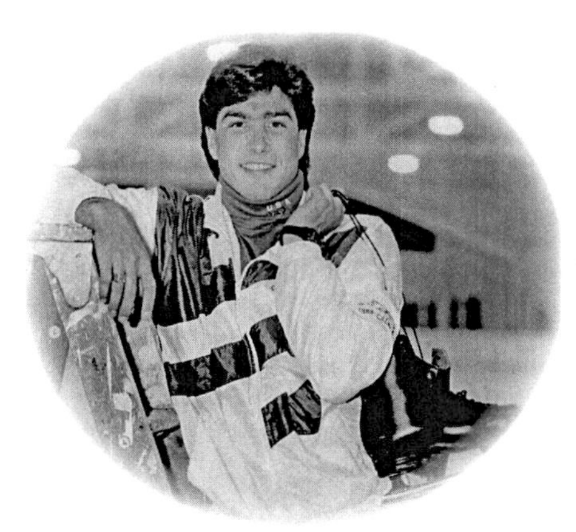

Retired from competitive skating, venturing into my teaching career at the University of Delaware Training Center.

Acknowledgments

Pam, Victoria, and me *(photo taken by my nephew, Greg Bodwell)*

Writing a book takes lots of time and thought to make it just right. I want to thank my wife, Pam, and daughter, Victoria, for being so patient and putting up with me while I was preoccupied during my book quest. I truly appreciate both of your input and suggestions. You always help put things in perspective and keep me grounded.

To be the best at whatever you pursue, you can't do it alone. Through my seventeen-plus years of skating, a lot of people helped shape me into a better athlete and stronger person. I am very grateful to all my coaches and choreographers for their inspirational tips and strong, disciplinary commands. Your kind, caring, and sincere tutelage helped me believe in myself and gave me the confidence that I could achieve anything!

My last ten years of competitive skating were solely in ice dancing. It takes two to tango, so I send heartfelt thanks to all my skating partners: Judy Ferris, for taking the chance to skate with me right after my knee surgery. We won our first national title within six months of skating together. Wow! You were great. The next four years, when I began allowing myself to consider becoming one of the country's top skaters, could not have been achieved without Lisa Spitz. We had our moments, but the best was making the 1984 Olympic team with you. Many times over, with great memories attached, thanks for being you. Then it came time for my final push to become one of the best skaters in the world. Two national championship titles, a fifth-ranked spot in the Worlds, and my second trip to the Olympics all came with the help of Suzy Semanick. Your eagerness to succeed and your talent is exquisite. Thanks for igniting the fire.

My love and gratitude goes to my family, near and far. You were always supportive–whether you came to my competitions or shows, sent letters of praise and gratitude, or prayed to help me through, you buoyed me up. From phone calls to letters to photos of me skating displayed in their homes, I always knew my grandparents were proud of their grandson. I wish they could hold and read this book. I guess I'll have to take one to heaven so they can read it there.

Life would be boring without friends. I am fortunate to have built friendships with people I met through skating and outside of skating. I'm lucky to have met you and am grateful you somehow found me interesting enough to be your friend.

Being a skater and a performer would not be the same without fans. When I was in the limelight, you showed me your appreciation in many ways. Thank you for being so supportive. I hope you find this book fun to read and inspirational.

When a kid starts out and then decides to pursue competitive skating, it is the United States Figure Skating Association that makes it possible for dreams to come true. Without the USFA, skating at national, international, Worlds and Olympic Events could not happen. My sincere thanks to the USFA for helping me achieve my Olympic dreams.

To my writer Diane Cook, who took my idea of writing a book and brought it to life. Your creativity and cleverness seemed to flow, word to word. The time we spent on the phone over the years has now come to a close. I hope you have continued success in the years ahead. Thank you so much for taking on my project.

To my publisher, Candy Abbott, with Fruitbearer Publishing, LLC. The opportunity to work with you was destined from the day we met at the Delaware Christian Writers Conference in 2006. You took an idea I had for the cover of the book and made a masterpiece. The advice and help you have given me is indescribable. I would describe your character as sincere and kind and am blessed to have you as my publisher.

About Scott Gregory

Scott was born in 1959 near his hometown, Skaneateles, in central New York, where he first encountered skating on ice. He took his first lessons at the age of eleven. His parents, brother, and sister bid him farewell when he relocated to Brynmaur, PA, at 15 to pursue his skating career. After a year, he relocated to Buffalo, NY, in 1980 moved to Wilmington, DE, and now resides in Newark, DE.

He competed in ice dancing at the 1984 Winter Olympics with Eliza Spitz Luliano. He then paired with Suzanne Semanick Schurman, with whom he won the gold medal at the U.S. Figure Skating Championships twice, ranked fifth in the Worlds (serving as a World team member seven consecutive times), and competed at the Olympics in 1988, placing sixth. Scott retired from competitive skating at twenty-eight due to back injuries. After graduating from two New York high schools, Skaneateles and Amherst Central, he gathered credits from Buffalo State, Philadelphia College of Arts, and the University of Delaware. In essence, he gained a master's degree in skating from his eight-year amateur pursuits. He has coached local, national, and international skaters, including Tara Lapinski from the ages of six and twelve, who went on to win the 1998 Winter Olympic gold medal in women's figure skating at the age of fifteen.

He has been married to Pam since 1995. Their daughter, Victoria, was born in 1998. Snappy, their turtle, came to live with them when Victoria was in third grade; he was the size of a quarter and is now the size of a softball. They also have a yellow English Lab named Polly that thinks she's still a puppy, even though she passed the six-year mark a while ago.

Ever since the 1988 Olympics, Scott has entertained the idea of writing a book to inspire people on how to overcome adversities. Then, in 2006, he attended a writers' conference. From that time on, he describes the journey as "long and grueling but exciting." Stay tuned . . . he even has ideas for one or more sequels to *Champion Mindset*.

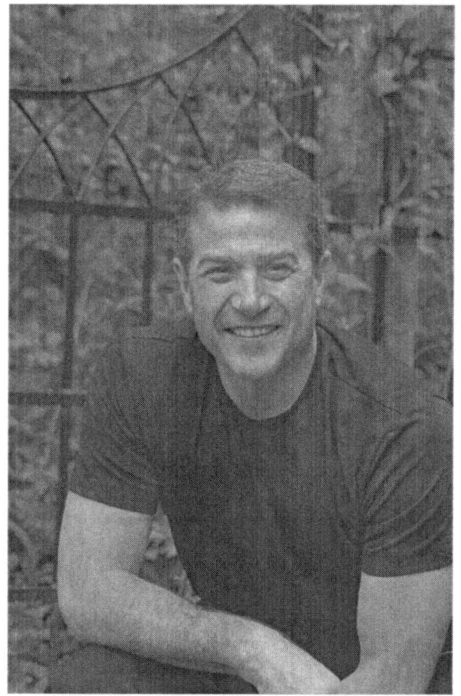

Photo by Diana Deluca (www.DianaDelucaPhotography.com)

Champion Mindset

Refusing to Give Up Your Dreams

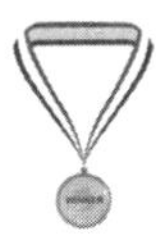

Thank you for reading my book. Through the years I've had the privilege of working with young athletes, guiding them through their own unique challenges as they learned to embrace the champion mindset. Are you eager for advice or do you have questions? Are you facing challenges or have you been through some? I would love to hear from you. Visit my website where you can connect with me through my blog. Need a speaker? Want an autograph? I would be honored. Looking forward to hearing from you.

www.ScottGregoryOlympian.com

Bulk discounts for fund-raisers
available through the publisher

Fruitbearer Publishing, LLC
P.O. Box 777 • Georgetown, DE 19947
(302) 856-6649 • FAX (302) 856-7742
www.fruitbearer.com • info@fruitbearer.com

Breinigsville, PA USA
24 October 2010
247965BV00001B/1/P
9 781886 068414